THE CARDIAC PATIENT

NURSING INTERVENTIONS

Editor

STEPHEN O'CONNOR
BSc, MA, RGN, CertFEd

Lecturer in Medical Nursing
University of Southampton and Acute Medical Directorate
Southampton University Hospitals NHS Trust
Southampton
UK

 Mosby

London Baltimore Bogotá Boston Buenos Aires Caracas Carlsbad, CA Chicago Madrid Mexico City Milan Naples, FL New York Philadelphia St. Louis
Sydney Tokyo Toronto Wiesbaden

Publisher:	Griselda Campbell
Project Manager:	Louise Cook
Production:	Joseph Lynch
Index:	Nina Boyd
Design:	Judith Gauge
Cover Design:	Lara Last
Illustrations:	Jenni Miller
	Lynda Payne

Copyright © 1995 Times Mirror International Publishers Limited.
Published in 1995 by Mosby, an imprint of Times Mirror International Publishers Limited.
Printed and bound in the UK by J.W. Arrowsmith Ltd., Bristol.
ISBN 0 7234 1916 7

For full details of all Times Mirror International Publishers Limited titles please write to: Times Mirror International Publishers Limited, Lynton House, 7–12 Tavistock Square, London WCIH 9LB, UK.

CONTENTS

CONTRIBUTORS

Maureen Coombs SRN, DipN (Lond), BSc (Hons), PGDipEd, ENB 100, 124. Senior Nurse/Service Delivery Unit Manager, Intensive Care Unit, John Radcliffe Hospital, Oxford.

Janet Dean BA (Hons), DipN, RGN. Lecturer/Practitioner in Medical Nursing, Southampton University College of Nursing and Midwifery, Southampton.

Robert Hall RGN, ENB 249, 998, DPSN. Senior Nurse, Cardiac Rehabilitation, St George's Hospital, London.

Jan Heath RGN, ENB 100, CertEd. Resuscitation Training Officer, Southampton University Hospitals NHS Trust, Southampton.

Isabella Lally BNSc, RGN, SCM. Senior Clinical Nurse, Cardiothoracic Intensive Care, Southampton University Hospitals NHS Trust, Southampton.

Julie Pearce BSc, RGN, ENB 100. Senior Research Fellow (Intensive Care Nursing), University of Southampton, and Senior Nurse, Research and Practice Development, Intensive Care Unit, Southampton University Hospitals NHS Trust, Southampton.

David Thompson BSc, MA, PhD, RN, FRCN. Professor of Nursing Studies, Institute for Nursing Studies, University of Hull.

David Voegli BSc (Hons), RGN, PGCEA, RNT. Lecturer/Practitioner in Medical Nursing, Southampton University College of Nursing and Midwifery, Southampton.

PREFACE

The care of patients with cardiac disorders occurs in various settings in a modern general hospital. Traditionally, such care was delivered in acute medical wards but the advent of coronary care units (CCUs) rapidly took over this provision. This shift in care provision quickly lead to specialised nursing staff who dealt solely with cardiac patients, usually those with myocardial infarctions, in a clinical setting designed for such care. However, even though this progression occurred in many areas, the care of cardiac patients was not entirely given over to specialist areas. Many hospitals retained the practice of caring for coronary patients in acute medical wards along with other acute medical patients. The reasons for this lack of progression are difficult to identify. As a consequence of caring for coronary patients in acute medical wards instead of CCUs more staff are involved with coronary patients and an ongoing programme of education and training is required because of the high levels of staff turnover on acute medical wards.

This book began as an exercise in ongoing clinical updating for junior staff at the Acute Medical Unit, Southampton University Hospitals NHS Trust. At the time of the design of the course, the unit consisted of six wards of 30 beds each. Each ward admitted casualties and general practitioner admissions on a daily rotation and there was no specialist CCU. The course was designed to meet the needs of junior staff, mostly newly qualified or with minimal experience in acute medicine, who care for acutely ill coronary patients. This course was developed over a period of several years and was continuously evaluated. This book reflects the content of that course, with additional chapters on subjects not covered in the course.

The audience for the book is therefore the junior nurse in acute medicine. However, the needs of these nurses are not dissimilar to other nurses in allied clinical areas. The nurse in an acute care-of-the-elderly ward will undoubtedly encounter a similar caseload as that of a nurse in general medicine. The nurse who is working on an intensive care or coronary care ward who has not yet undertaken the respective ENB course will also find in this book valuable information at an appropriate level. The advent of Project 2000 and especially the Adult Branch has augmented the knowledge base of students as academic standards are raised; hence the content of this book will be of great value to senior Adult Branch students who may be revisiting the subjects of acute medical care or care of the elderly. Together with the growth in Project 2000 there has been a concomitant growth in undergraduate courses. Such courses, whether traditional or Project 2000 style, require the student who is caring in the areas of acute medicine and care of the elderly to be cognisant of the care of acutely ill coronary patients. In the case of both these groups of students, the contents of this book will inform their clinical experience and create a firm basis from which competent clinical practice can develop on qualification.

The book is divided into three sections. Section 1 – Foundations of patient care – seeks to lay out the groundwork upon which the care of coronary patients is based, and includes normal anatomy and physiology of cardiovascular system since knowledge of this system is central to the understanding of the patient's problems. The majority of medical interventions, almost by definition, include the use of pharmacological agents. A sound knowledge of these is therefore essential to an understanding of the patient's treatment. Many cardiac drugs are available for prescription by doctors and prescription patterns continually alter as different agents become available. Similarly, certain cardiac drugs go out of fashion and are no longer commonly used. This chapter therefore looks at the key cardiac agents that have stood the test of time and will be in use in all circumstances. However, more importantly, the chapter deals with the subject by addressing the actions of groups or types of drugs and examples of that group are used. Cardiac patients can now be subject to a plethora of investigations both minor and major, the nurse must have a sound knowledge of these tests and their implications for the patient. The nurse's ability to observe the patient and interpret what is seen and heard is the central focus of the nurse's intervention with cardiac patients. The ability to interpret this knowledge provides the nurse with the foresight to be aware of what to report and when to intervene.

Section 2 – Immediate patient care – deals with various patient presentations commonly seen in the acute care of coronary patients. These chapters are designed to stand alone but with readers having an understanding of Section 1. There is therefore some overlap in the content in terms of the interventions and treatments. The chapters in this section discuss the common features of coronary illness that are confronted frequently. It is these clinical features, rather than specific medical conditions such as myocardial infarction or left ventricular failure, that are the focus of the team's activity. The commonest physical features, chest pain and low cardiac output, are dealt with first, followed by key complications of coronary disease; these have significant implications for all aspects of the nurses care. The next three chapters on bradycardia, tachycardia and left ventricular failure and acute pulmonary oedema, require the nurse to be alert in the recognition of these complications and a sound understanding is required. All these chapters have been addressed in such a fashion as to enable the nurse to make informed choices and to be aware of the choice since a coronary event carries with it a strong emotional load. The fear of death in coronary patients is a common phenomenon and the nurse's ability to deal with these feelings is central to the patient's well being, both on admission and throughout the hospital stay. In coronary care, cardiac arrest occurs despite the best endeavours of the team. A sound and up-to-date knowledge of resuscitation procedures is therefore a prerequisite.

Section 3 – Ongoing patient care – reflects the fact that from the earliest opportunity, the nurse is involved in the preparation of the patient for discharge and the return, where appropriate, to a full life. To this end, the nurse must be aware of the patient's need for education and the principles of cardiac rehabilitation. In this section, these are discussed fully to provide the nurse with both the knowledge and the confidence to commence educational programmes and, once the acute stage can be deemed to be over, to prepare the patient for a programme of rehabilitation that will continue well after discharge from hospital. This section is seen by all those concerned with the book as containing information that is as vital to the patient's eventual well being as any other intervention that the nurse may undertake.

Stephen O'Connor
Southampton
1994

SECTION 1:

FOUNDATIONS OF PATIENT CARE

1.

NORMAL ANATOMY AND PHYSIOLOGY OF THE HEART AND CARDIOVASCULAR SYSTEM

The functioning of the human body is dependent on the collective functioning of all cells. Each cell requires a stable internal environment with a constant supply of oxygen and nutrients and removal of the waste products of metabolism. The circulatory and lymphatic systems work to perform these functions.

The purpose of this chapter is to provide a general description of the cardiovascular system, including the structure and function of the heart, a basic description of the electrical and mechanical events occurring during the cardiac cycle, and an overview of the factors involved in the regulation of cardiac output.

The cardiovascular system is essentially a closed transport system for nutritive and waste materials, hormones, heat energy and defence cells. It provides a continuous supply of oxygenated blood to metabolising tissues. Blood is driven around the circulatory system by pressure developed as a result of the mechanical pumping action of the heart. It is also a dynamic system and it is able to adjust and maintain blood flow to tissues according to metabolic demand. The metabolic demand will vary greatly based on the level of physical activity, e.g. at rest, during sleep, moderate and vigorous exercise, or changes in physiological state, such as during pregnancy. Blood flow to the vital organs such as the brain and heart has priority. Tissues that do not receive an adequate blood flow quickly demonstrate signs of ischaemia.

There is a finite volume of blood, therefore the adjustments made are to cardiac output and the distribution of blood to areas with a higher metabolic need, e.g. skeletal muscle during physical activity. These changes are primarily under the influence of the autonomic nervous system, circulating hormones, and local factors such as changes in pH and body temperature.

The main functions of the cardiovascular support system are as follows:

- Delivery of oxygen, hormones and defence cells to all body tissues.
- Removal of carbon dioxide and the end products of metabolism from tissues and delivery to the appropriate organs for breakdown and elimination, e.g. the lungs, liver and kidneys.
- Dissipation of heat away from active tissue and its redistribution around the body to maintain normal body temperature.

GENERAL DESCRIPTION OF THE CARDIOVASCULAR SYSTEM

The cardiovascular system is essentially a closed transport system. It is composed of two major subdivisions: a pulmonary circulation (carrying blood to and from the lungs) and a systemic circulation (carrying blood to all areas of the body and bringing it back to the heart). Each includes a pump (right and left sides of the heart) and a circuit of vascular tubes (the arteries, arterioles, capillaries and veins). The arteries and veins are elastic tubes that essentially provide a connection between the lungs, tissues and heart. The capillary network of each circuit provides a specialised exchange surface for the movement of gases, nutrients and waste products. Exchange occurs by diffusion of substances down concentration and pressure gradients, i.e. from areas of high concentration or pressure to areas of lower concentration or pressure.

The main purpose of the pulmonary circulation is to bring desaturated blood within close proximity of the oxygen-rich alveolar air. The blood leaves the right side of the heart through the pulmonary artery which bifurcates and supplies each lung. The arteries divide on several levels, ultimately forming arterioles and enter the pulmonary capillary beds. Blood saturated with oxygen then returns to the left side of the heart via the venules and four pulmonary veins.

The systemic circulation supplies the body tissues with oxygen and nutrients. All the blood for the systemic circulation leaves the left side of the heart via the aorta. This large artery divides into smaller branches and blood is delivered to all tissues and organs. The arteries continue to divide into arterioles, which then enter the capillary beds where the exchange of gases, nutrients and waste products occurs. Blood leaves the capillary network via venules which join and form larger vessels known as veins. The veins unite to form two large veins – the inferior vena cava (from the lower portion of the body) and the superior vena cava (from the head and arms), which return desaturated blood to the right side of the heart.

There are several parallel circuits within the systemic circulation. Normally there is only one capillary bed for each branch of a circuit; however, there are some instances where there are two capillary beds, one following another, i.e. in series. For example, a proportion of the blood supplied to the liver is venous blood coming directly from the gastrointestinal tract and spleen via the hepatic portal vein. This arrangement enables the digested and absorbed substances from the gut to be transported directly to the liver, where many of the body's metabolic requirements are synthesised.

The force required to move the blood through the blood vessels in both circulations is provided by the heart. The systemic circulation is much larger than the pulmonary circulation and offers more resistance to blood flow. Therefore the pressure generated by the left side of the heart is much greater than that of the right side of the heart. The volume of blood pumped through the pulmonary circulation in a given period of time must equal the volume pumped through the systemic circulation. In a normal resting adult, the average volume of blood pumped simultaneously is approximately 5 litres/minute. During heavy work or exercise, the volume of blood pumped by the heart can increase up to 25 litres/minute.

THE HEART: LOCATION AND STRUCTURE

The heart lies within the mediastinum, which is the central part of the thorax lying between the two pleural sacs, which themselves contain the lungs. The mediastinum extends from the sternum to the vertebral column and contains all the thoracic organs except the lungs (Fig. 1-1). The heart is shaped like a blunt cone and is about the size of a closed fist, i.e. 12 cm long, 9 cm wide at its broadest point, and 6 cm thick. Approximately two-thirds of the mass of the heart lies to the left of the body's midline.

The apex is formed by the tip of the left ventricle, and projects inferiorly, anteriorly and to the left. The left border is formed almost entirely by the left ventricle. The superior border, where the great vessels enter and leave the heart, is formed by the atria. The base of the heart projects superiorly, posteriorly and to the right; it is formed mostly by the left atrium. The right border is formed by the right atrium, and the inferior border is formed by the right ventricle and a small part of the left ventricle.

The heart is made up of four chambers, which consist mainly of muscle tissue. The right and left atria receive blood from the veins, whereas the right and left ventricles pump blood out into the arterial systems. The entry and exit points of the ventricles are guarded by valves.

The heart is enclosed and held in place by the pericardium. This is an interesting structure that consists of two parts: an outer fibrous layer and an inner serous pericardium. The outer fibrous layer provides a tough protective membrane around

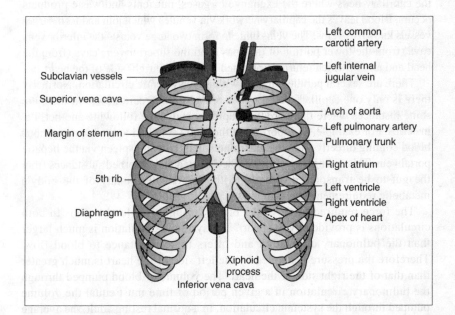

Fig. 1-1 Location of the heart and associated blood vessels in the thoracic cavity. Adapted from Hincliffe, S., Montague, S. (1988). *Physiology for Nursing Practice*, Balliere Tindall, London, p.320.

the heart and anchors it in the mediastinum by attachments to the great vessels, the diaphragm and the sternal chest wall; the inner serous pericardium is a thinner, more delicate membrane and consists of a double layer of epithelium. A small amount of fluid secreted by the epithelial cells is present between the two layers and prevents friction between the membranes as the heart moves and holds the serous pericardial layers together. The space occupied by the pericardial fluid is a potential space called the pericardial cavity.

An inflammation of the pericardium is known as pericarditis and is often associated with a pericardial friction rub, which can be heard on auscultation of the pericardial area. A build up of pericardial fluid or extensive bleeding into the pericardium, if untreated, is a life-threatening condition. The fibrous pericardium is not able to stretch and therefore the heart becomes compressed. This compression is known as cardiac tamponade and can result in cardiac failure.

The connective tissue between the pericardium and the myocardium contains blood vessels, nerves and the autonomic ganglia.

Heart wall

The wall of the heart is divided into three layers: the epicardium (external layer), the myocardium (middle layer), and the endocardium (inner layer). The epicardium is formed by the visceral layer of the serous pericardium. The myocardium is cardiac muscle tissue and forms the bulk of the walls of each of the chambers. The myocardium of the left ventricle is much thicker than that of the right; this enables the left ventricle to develop much greater pressure when it contracts. The myocardium consists of two types of cells: contractile (atrial and ventricular muscle) and conducting tissue [e.g. in the sinoatrial (SA) node, atrioventricular (AV) node, bundle of His and Purkinje cells].

Both types of cells develop embryologically from the same precursor cells and consequently have common features. The conducting tissue still possesses some contractile proteins, even though these cells do not play a part in developing pressures in the heart. Additionally, the atrial and ventricular muscle has some similarities with the electrical properties of the conducting cells. The nature and properties of the contractile and conduction cells will be described on page 9.

The endocardium is a thin layer of endothelium overlying a thin layer of connective tissue. It lines the inside of the myocardium and is continuous with the endothelial lining of the large blood vessels of the heart (Fig. 1-2).

Chambers of the heart

The interior of the heart is divided into four chambers. The upper two chambers are the right and left atria. The atria are separated by a partition called the interatrial septum. A prominent feature of this septum is an ovalis depression, the fossa ovalis, which corresponds to the site of the foramen ovale, which is an opening within the septum of the fetal heart. Failure or partial failure of the foramen ovale closing results in an atrial septal defect.

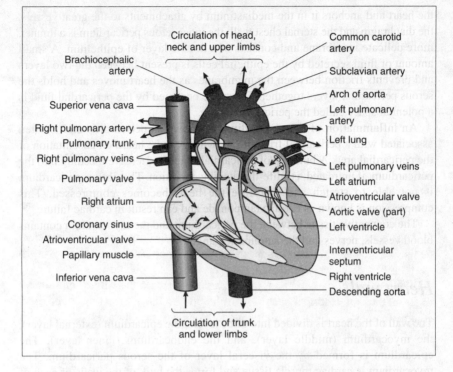

Fig. 1-2 Structure of the heart and direction of blood flow. Adapted from Hincliffe, S., Montague, S. (1988). *Physiology for Nursing Practice*, Balliere Tindall, London, p.321.

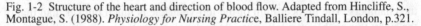

The two lower chambers are the right and left ventricles. They are separated by an interventricular septum. Again ventricular septal defects may arise when complete development of the interventricular septum is interrupted.

The atria and ventricles are separated by a dense, fibrous structure into which the muscle cells are inserted. Openings in this band of tissue, between the atria and the ventricles, are guarded by valves, consisting of flaps of connective tissue. There are valves also at the exit points from the ventricles into the pulmonary artery and aorta.

Externally, a groove known as the coronary sulcus separates the atria from the ventricles. It encircles the heart and houses the coronary sinus and the circumflex branch of the left coronary artery. The anterior and posterior interventricular sulci separate the right and left ventricles externally.

The thickness of the four chambers varies according to the pressures generated within them. The atria are thin-walled because a larger percentage of ventricular filling is not dependent on atrial contraction. The ventricles fill with blood during diastole, this is a passive process aided by gravity and a reduced pressure created by the expanding ventricles. Atrial contraction contributes the last 30% of ventricular filling and therefore a relatively small amount of the work is involved.

The right ventricle has a thicker layer of myocardium and is capable of generating moderate pressures needed to overcome the resistance offered by the pulmonary circulation. The left ventricular wall is made up a thick layer of myocardium and is capable of generating higher pressures needed to drive the blood around the systemic circulation.

The heart valves

The valves between the atria and the ventricles are the mitral (left side of the heart) and tricuspid valve (right side of the heart). The tricuspid valve is made up of three cusps or flaps of fibrous tissue that grow out of the walls of the heart and are covered with endocardium. The mitral or bicuspid valve has two cusps, which work in the same way as the tricuspid valve.

The valves (Fig. 1-3) are attached to muscular projections (papillary muscles) on the ventricular walls by fibrous strands called chordae tendineae. These keep the flaps of the valves pointing in the direction of the blood flow.

When the ventricles contract, the pressure exerted on the valves forces them to close, thus preventing a back flow of blood into the atria. At the same time, contraction of the papillary muscles and tightening of the chordae tendineae help to prevent the valve from swinging upwards into the atrium.

The valves that lie between the ventricles and the major arteries are termed the semilunar valves because of their shape. They are the aortic and pulmonary valves. Both valves consist of three semilunar cusps attached by their convex margins to

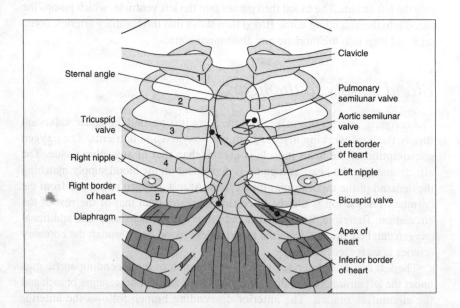

Fig. 1-3 Position of the heart valves. Large dots indicate where heart sounds caused by the respective heart valves are best heard. Adapted from Tortora, G.J., Anagnostakos, N.P. (1987). *Principles of Anatomy and Physiology*, Harper and Row Pub., New York, p.468.

the artery wall. The free borders of the cusps curve outwards and project into the opening inside the blood vessel. They are not tethered by cords of connective tissue, however, they ensure that blood flows in the correct direction, i.e. from the ventricles into the aorta and pulmonary artery.

Damage to the heart valves can disrupt the blood flow through the heart. Rheumatic fever, subacute bacterial endocarditis and arthrosclerotic changes are common causes of valvular damage. The damage causes stenosis or fusing of the valve tissue and narrowing of the opening through which the blood flows; damage to the edges of the cusps renders them incompetent and allows back flow or regurgitation of blood through the valve.

Stenosed or incompetent valves cause additional abnormal heart sounds on auscultation. The turbulent flow produces a murmur. Damaged valves decrease the efficiency of the heart as a pump and generally the heart has to work harder to achieve a satisfactory cardiac output, particularly during times of stress or exercise. The long-term effect may result in heart failure.

The great vessels of the heart

The right atrium receives blood from all parts of the body, except the lungs, via the superior vena cava, inferior vena cava and the coronary sinus, which drains blood from most vessels supplying the wall of the heart.

The right atrium delivers blood into the right ventricle, which pumps it into the pulmonary trunk. The pulmonary trunk divides into the left and right pulmonary arteries, each of which carries desaturated blood to the lungs.

Saturated blood returns to the heart via four pulmonary veins, which empty into the left atrium. The blood then passes into the left ventricle, which pumps the blood into the ascending aorta. Blood then flows into the coronary arteries, aortic arch and then into the thoracic and abdominal aorta.

Blood supply to the heart

The coronary arteries originate from the aorta just beyond the aortic valve and supply the hard-working myocardium with oxygen and nutrients. The oxygen consumption of the heart muscle is greater than that of any other tissue. The effectiveness of the heart as a pump is dependent on the blood supply matching the demand of the myocardium for oxygen. At rest, oxygen extraction from the coronary circulation is almost three times greater than that of the rest of the circulation. Therefore, when the demand for oxygen is increased, little additional oxygen can be extracted from the blood unless blood flow through the coronary arteries is increased.

The left coronary artery originates as a branch of the ascending aorta, runs under the left atrium, before dividing into the left anterior descending branch and the circumflex branch. The anterior descending branch follows the anterior interventricular sulcus and supplies blood to the anterior wall of the left ventricle and portions of the right ventricle. The circumflex branch supplies the left atrium and the posterior wall of the left ventricle.

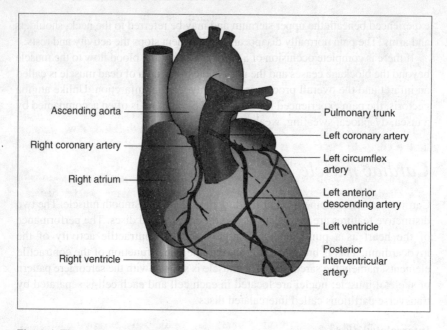

Fig. 1-4 The coronary circulation. Adapted from Hinchcliffe, S., Montague, S. (1988). *Physiology for Nursing Practice*, Balliere Tindall, London, p. 325.

The right coronary artery also originates as a branch of the ascending aorta. It supplies the right atrium and right ventricle and a portion of the left ventricle.

The coronary arteries (Fig. 1-4) lie on the surface of the heart and branches penetrate deep into the myocardium. Anastomoses between the branches of one coronary artery or between branches of different coronary arteries provide collateral circulation (alternative routes) so that all areas of the myocardium receive blood. When a major vessel is obstructed, blood will flow through the collateral vessels. Although the collaterals of the heart are quite small, the myocardium is able to survive as long as it receives at least 10–15% of its normal supply.

The blood flow through the coronary circulation is pulsatile. Resistance offered to blood flow is greater during systole, therefore blood flows more easily during ventricular diastole when the myocardium is relaxed. Venous blood drains either directly into the four chambers of the heart or flows into a venous drainage system. The venous blood from the left ventricle returns to the right atrium through the coronary sinus. Most of the venous blood from the right ventricle drains into the anterior cardiac veins into the right atrium.

Angina pectoris is often the first sign of an obstruction of the coronary arteries great enough to cause ischaemia of the heart muscle, particularly during stress and increased activity. The pain experienced results from the fact that myocardial oxygen demand is greater than the delivery of oxygen to the myocardium, i.e. coronary blood flow has not increased sufficiently to cope with the extra demand. The pain is usually experienced beneath the upper sternum and may be referred to the neck, shoulders and arms. The pain normally disappears if the patient stops the activity and rests.

If there is complete occlusion of a coronary artery, the blood flow to the muscle beyond the blockage ceases and the muscle dies. The area of dead muscle is called an infarct and the overall process is called myocardial infarction. Unlike angina pectoris, the pain experienced is not relieved by rest and is often accompanied by nausea, dyspnoea, sweating, weakness and fear.

Cardiac muscle

Cardiac muscle combines properties of both skeletal and smooth muscle. The two distinctive features are the striations and the intercalated discs. The performance of the heart as a pump depends largely on the contractile activity of the myocardium. This is brought about by the integrated function of the contractile elements, namely the sarcomere. The muscle is striated with the sarcomere pattern of skeletal muscle; nuclei are located in each cell and each cell is separated by transverse partitions called intercalated discs.

Intercalated discs
These are specialised cells that firmly link individual cells together. This creates a closely interwoven network of cells with a very low electrical resistance, allowing electrical activity to spread easily from cell to cell. The discs allow the cardiac muscle cells to work together as a functional unit, known as a syncytium.

Striations
The cells also have a striped (striated) appearance (Fig. 1-5). This is because the rod-like fibrils contain cross-striations of thick myosin and thin actin filaments. The fibrils are surrounded by numerous mitochondria which provide the source of energy required to produce contraction of the sarcomere.

The thick and thin filaments are interleaved, arranged in groups and divided by a structure called the 'z line'. This basic arrangement forms the sarcomere and is repeated many times to form a long myofibril. Each striated muscle cell contains bundles of myofibrils extending from one end of the cell to the other.

The distinctive pattern of light and dark arises because the places where the thick and thin filaments overlap (the 'A band') look different under an electron microscope from those where they do not (the 'I band').

The other distinctive features of cardiac muscle include the presence of many mitochondria, the sarcoplasmic reticulum and the T tubules. The mitochondria lie between the myofibrils and generate adenosine triphosphate (ATP), which provides energy for contraction to take place. The sarcoplasmic reticulum is more extensive in cardiac muscle and is interlaced between the myofibrils, acting as an important store of intracellular calcium. The T tubules consist of invaginations of the cell walls to form long, narrow tubes. These tubules transmit the electrical impulse deep into the interior of the cell.

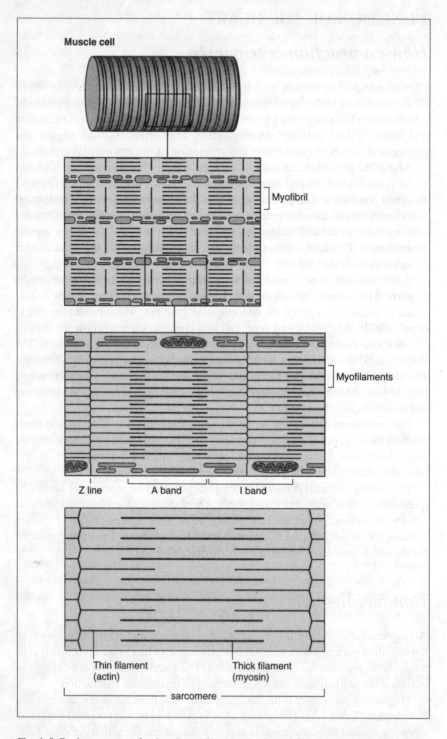

Fig. 1-5 Basic structure of striated muscle: organisation of filaments and fibrils within a cardiac muscle cell. Adapted from Rutishauser, S. (1994). *Physiology and Anatomy: A Basis for Nursing and Health Care*, Churchill Livingstone, Edinburgh, p. 391.

FUNCTION OF THE HEART

How contraction is triggered

Cardiac muscle, like smooth muscle, contracts and relaxes regularly. The source of the excitation is the conducting tissue, which generates action potentials, which in turn are transmitted to all myocardial cells. The electrical excitation and activities of cellular depolarisation and repolarisation trigger the mechanical events of contraction and relaxation of the myocardial muscle.

At rest, the myocardial cell is said to be polarised. This phenomenon is related to the properties of the cell membrane (sarcolemma), which creates a negative electrical potential within the cell because of the impermeability of the membrane to sodium ions and the relative difference in concentration of sodium ions outside (extracellular fluid) and inside (intracellular fluid) the cell. There is a greater concentration of sodium ions outside the cell in comparison with the concentration of sodium ions inside the cell.

When the cell is activated the sarcolemma ceases to be a barrier to the movement of sodium ions into the cell. The sodium channels open to allow a rapid influx of sodium ions down the concentration gradient, which causes the cell to depolarise. In the depolarised state, calcium channels open to allow the flow of calcium ions from the extracellular fluid and the sarcoplasmic reticulum. The calcium ions bind to troponin, which displaces the troponin–tropomyosin complex. This in turn exposes the attachment sites of the myosin and actin filaments causing them to join and form actomyosin. This brings about contraction of the sarcomere and muscle contraction occurs.

The subsequent detachment of the filaments and relaxation of the muscle fibres requires the presence of magnesium ions. Calcium ions are pumped back into the sarcoplasm and transported out of the cell, the inhibitory effect of the troponin–tropomyosin complex is established and relaxation occurs.

The resting potential is restored by repolarisation. This is an active metabolic process occurring within the sarcolemma. The sodium ions are extruded from the cell by the sodium pump, until the difference in ionic concentrations of sodium between the intracellular and extracellular fluids is achieved. The energy required for the whole process is released by the hydrolysis of ATP.

Conducting cells

All myocardial cells have the properties of conduction and contraction; however, the modified pacemaker cells also have automaticity that other myocardial cells have lost in the process of differentiation. The pacemaker cells are capable of initiating the activation of the whole process of myocardial contraction.

The normal pacemaker is the SA node, these cells have the fastest inherent rate and rhythm (Table 1.1). The sinoatrial cells reach an action potential before all other myocardial cells, this tends to suppress the pacemaker activity of other cells. However, if the SA node fails to bring about activation, then the AV node, which has the next fastest inherent discharge rate, will take over as pacemaker.

Table 1.1 The inherent rate of the conducting cells of the heart.

Conducting cell	Inherent rate (beats/min)
Sino atrial node	150
Atrioventricular node	40–60
Bundle of His	30–40
Purkinje cells	20–30
Ventricular myocardial cell	20–30

Cardiac events (electrical): conduction of the impulse

The conduction system of the heart is shown in Fig. 1–6. The impulse generated by the cells of the SA node, which is situated in the wall of the right atrium and to the right of the superior vena caval orifice, spreads across the right and left atrial muscle. The impulse reaches the AV node situated in the right atrium above the tricuspid valve and just to the right of the interatrial septum. After a delay at the AV node, mainly from the slow movement of calcium ions, the impulse travels down the bundle of His, right and left bundle branches and into the Purkinje system.

The bundle of His passes horizontally to the left from the AV node, pierces the membranous intraventricular septum and divides into the right bundle branch and the left anterior and posterior branches. The branches pass down on either side of the interventricular septum and finally divide into the Purkinje network of fibres, which proceed vertically to the surface of the heart from the endocardium to the epicardium.

The activation process arising in the SA node sweeps to the left, anteriorly and downwards across the atria causing the muscle fibres to contract, bringing about atrial systole. These events are reflected as the P wave on the electrocardiogram (ECG). The delay of entry of the impulses to the ventricles by the AV node ensures that enough time for ventricular filling to take place is available by convention this is called the P–R segment (Fig. 1-7).

The cells of the bundle of His and the Purkinje tissue are specialised for rapid conduction of the impulse. It is only when the process reaches the terminal Purkinje fibres beneath the endocardium, that the main mass of ventricular muscle begins to be activated and sufficient voltage changes occur to give deflections in the conventional surface ECG.

The first part of the ventricles to be activated is the ventricular septum, the main bulk of the septum is made up of muscle that is embryologically and functionally part of the left ventricle. The process of activation begins on the left side of the septum and spreads towards the right, producing a deflection labelled 'Q deflection'. This is quickly followed by activation of the main mass of ventricular muscle. The left ventricle is larger than the right and normally dominates the electrical process, this produces the 'R deflection', followed by an 'S deflection' as the right ventricle is activated. The whole process of ventricular activation is known as the QRS complex.

During the next stage, there is little difference in potential across the cell membrane and the ECG remains at the base line (ST segment). The recovery process of the ventricles begins during this interval and there is a final deflection of the 'T wave' corresponding to ventricular repolarisation; the muscle remains in diastole.

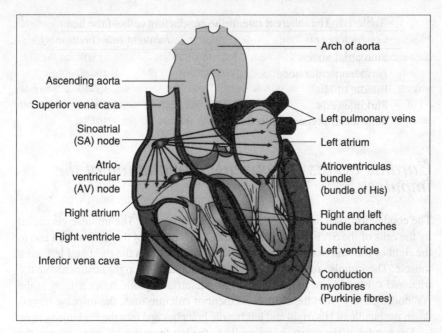

Fig, 1–6 Conduction system of the heart. Adapted from Tortora, G.J., Anagnostakos, N.P. (1987). *Principles of Anatomy and Physiology,* Harper and Row Pub., New York, p. 468.

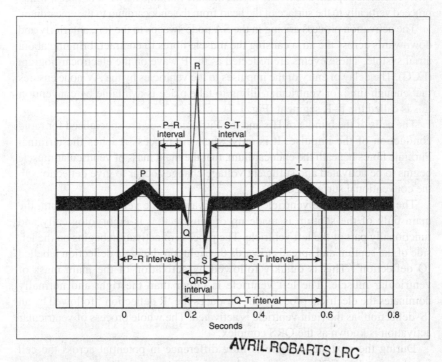

AVRIL ROBARTS LRC

Fig. 1–7 Normal electrocardiograph of a single heart beat. Adapted from Tortora, G.J., Anagnostakos, N.P. (1987). *Principles of Anatomy and Physiology*, Harper and Row Pub., New York, p. 468.

In general, recovery is much slower than the activation process. Atrial recovery (repolarisation) is not normally evident since it is masked by the QRS complex. However, it may be visible as a slight depression in the ST segment when the rate is fast. The pathway of recovery (repolarisation) in the ventricle is almost the reverse of activation, spreading inwards from the epicardium. The T wave is normally similar in direction to the QRS complex because the underlying electrical changes in the heart are also opposite to those producing activation.

The electrocardiograph

The electrical activity generated by the activation of the conducting cells and the muscle cells is relatively small. These electrical events spread to the surface of the body where the potential difference can be measured using skin electrodes and a galvanometer. The activity is then recorded as an electrocardiograph (ECG).

The shape, side and direction (upright or inverted) of a wave or complex is known as the configuration. When monitoring a patient, the configuration will depend on where the electrodes are placed on the chest and the channel selected for monitoring. However, ischaemic heart disease, electrolyte disturbances and dysrhythmias will affect the configuration of the complex and the 12-lead ECG using standardised leads is an important adjunct to diagnosis.

Neural and hormonal control

The rate of discharge of the SA node can take place spontaneously in the absence of any hormonal or neural influences. However, in reality it is under the continuous influence of both. The nerves of the heart are derived from the vagus (Xth cranial nerve) and the cervical ganglionated sympathetic chain, which forms the superior, middle and inferior cardiac nerves.

The depolarisation of pacemaker cells is slightly more complex than that of the other myocardial cells in that there is a slow depolarisation (prepotential) occurring prior to an action potential. There is a gradual rise in the resting potential produced by an increasing influx of sodium ions into the cell throughout the resting phase until a threshold potential is reached. The threshold potential triggers the opening of the sodium channels and a rapid influx of sodium ions bringing about an action potential and depolarisation (Fig. 1-8).

The rate of influx of sodium ions and the decrease in the permeability of the membrane to potassium ions during the prepotential phase is affected by the presence of noradrenaline from sympathetic nerve endings and acetylcholine from the parasympathetic fibres.

An increase in sympathetic tone produces more noradrenaline, which increases the prepotential gradient, i.e. the rate of influx of sodium and calcium ions increases and the threshold potential and action potential is reached more quickly. Repolarisation occurs rapidly, therefore the number of impulses per minute generated by the SA node is increased.

An increase in parasympathetic tone slows down the heart rate by slowing the rate of influx of sodium ions during the prepotential phase so that the threshold potential is reached more slowly. It is thought that acetylcholine also increases the threshold potential required to activate the action potential. In the resting state, the parasympathetic influence is dominant.

Other factors also influence the heart rate. Adrenaline, a sympathetic mediator of the adrenal medulla will have the same effect as noradrenaline, stimulating the beta receptors, increasing the heart rate and force of contraction. Changes in pH and body temperature will also affect the heart rate.

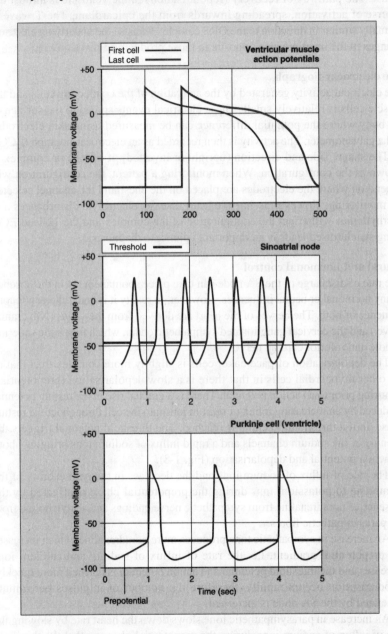

Fig. 1–8 The action potential. Top, ventricular muscle cell; middle, sino atrial node cell; bottom, Purkinje cell. Adapted from Rutishauser, S. (1994). *Physiology and Anatomy: A Basis for Mursing and Health Care*, Churchill Livingstone, Edinburgh, p.393.

Cardiac events (mechanical)

Two phenomena control the movement of blood through the heart: the opening and closing of the valves and the contraction and relaxation of the myocardium. Both of these activities occur without direct stimulation from the autonomic nervous system. The valves are controlled by pressure changes in each heart chamber, while contraction of the cardiac muscle is brought about by pacemaker activity of the SA node and the conduction system.

Blood flows from an area of higher pressure to an area of lower pressure. The pressure developed in a heart chamber is inversely proportional to its size. For example, if the chamber size decreases as with contraction of the ventricles, the pressure inside the ventricles will increase.

Blood flow through the heart and circulation is related to pressure differences (the higher the pressure the larger the flow), and inversely related to resistance (the greater the resistance the smaller the flow). In the circulation, pressure is generated by contraction of the heart, and resistance to flow is created by the size of the blood vessels (arteries and arterioles) and the viscosity of the blood.

The term systole refers to the phase of contraction; diastole is the phase of relaxation. A cardiac cycle consists of a systole and diastole of both atria, followed by systole and diastole of both ventricles. The cardiac cycle is shown in Fig. 1-9.

Atrial systole (contraction)

Blood flows continuously from the superior and inferior vena cavae and coronary sinus into the right atrium and from the pulmonary veins into the left atrium. Approximately 70% of blood flows passively from the atrium into the ventricles prior to atrial contraction. Contraction of the atria forces the remaining 30% blood into the ventricles.

Ventricular filling

When the ventricles are contracting, the mitral and tricuspid valves are closed and atrial pressure increases as the atria fill with blood. Once ventricular systole is over, ventricular pressure falls and the higher pressure within the atria pushes open the mitral and tricuspid valves and blood fills the ventricles.

The major part of ventricular filling occurs as soon as the valves open, there is a period of rapid filling, followed by a period where blood continually entering the atria passes straight into the ventricles; the last third of ventricular filling occurs as a result of atrial contraction.

Ventricular systole (contraction)

The beginning of ventricular contraction coincides with the first heart sound. There is an abrupt rise in ventricular pressure, which causes the mitral and tricuspid valves to close (lubb). The first 0.05 seconds of ventricular systole is known as isovolumetric contraction because the volume is constant until the pressure in the ventricles is greater than the pressure in the arterial system; it is at this point that the aortic and pulmonary valves open. Blood then flows from the ventricles into the respective arteries. This is called the ejection period and lasts for about 0.25 seconds,

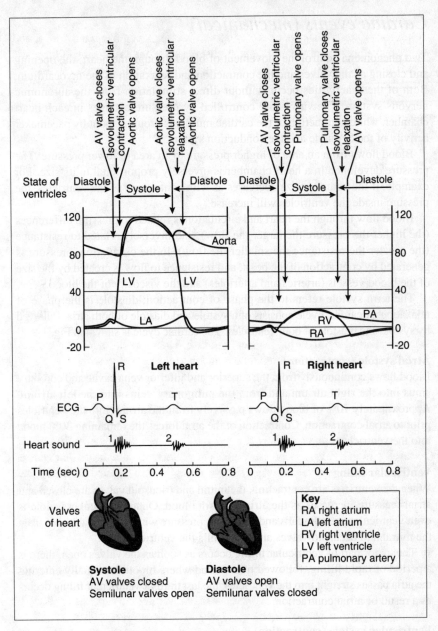

Fig. 1–9 The cardiac cycle. Adapted from Hinchcliffe, S., Montague, S. (1988). *Physiology for Nursing Practice*, Balliere Tindall, London, p.345.

until the aortic and pulmonary valves close. The volume of blood pumped out the ventricles during each ejection is known as the stroke volume and normally is about 50% of the content of the ventricles; the ventricles do not empty completely.

Ventricular diastole (relaxation)

At the end of ventricular systole, the ventricles suddenly begin to relax. The period between the opening of the mitral and tricuspid valves and the closing of the aortic and pulmonary valves is called isovolumetric relaxation. It is characterised by a dramatic fall in ventricular pressure without a change in ventricular volume.

The higher pressures within the arterial systems causes the blood to flow back towards the ventricles, this results in the closure of the semilunar valves. The closure of the aortic valve produces a brief rise in arterial pressure (dicrotic notch) and the second heart sound (dubb). The average heart rate at rest is 75 beats/minute and each cardiac cycle requires 0.8 seconds. When the heart rate is faster than normal, the relaxation period is shortened.

REGULATION OF CARDIAC OUTPUT

The amount of blood ejected from the heart per minute is determined by the heart rate and the stroke volume, i.e. the volume of blood ejected from a ventricle during each systole. Thus, cardiac output equals heart rate multiplied by stroke volume. In the healthy individual, heart rate at rest can range from 60–80 beats/minute to 180 beats/minute during vigorous exercise. The stroke volume can range from 70 ml at rest to 120 ml during physical exercise. Therefore the cardiac output can range from between 5 litres/minute to a maximum over 20 litres/minute.

Heart rate is determined by the activity of the SA node. The SA node is innervated by both the parasympathetic and sympathetic nervous systems. The autonomic control of the heart rate is the result of opposing sympathetic (stimulatory) and parasympathetic (inhibitory) influences. Sensory information from the baroreceptors (pressure receptors) found within the carotid sinus and aortic arch monitors arterial pressure and sends information to the cardiac centres (cardio-acceleratory and cardio-inhibitory centres) within the medulla oblongata.

An increase in arterial pressure will stimulate the baroceptors, which will inhibit the cardio-acceleratory centre, thus reducing sympathetic tone. It will also stimulate the cardio-inhibitory centre, which will increase parasympathetic tone. The net result is a decrease in heart rate and force of contraction, a decrease in cardiac output and arterial pressure.

Other factors that affect the heart rate by their direct action on the SA node include body temperature and circulating hormones from the thyroid gland. Any increase in body temperature will increase the heart rate. Similarly, if the body is cooled, as in hypothermia, the heart rate will fall.

An increase in activity of the thyroid gland that results in the increase of circulating thyroxine (T_4) and tri-iodothyronine (T_3) increases the heart rate. However, the cardiac centre in the medulla is under the influence of many factors. The most important are the higher centres: emotional stress increases the heart rate. Sensory nerves will have a variable effect on heart rate; slight pain will increase heart rate, whereas severe pain may bring about a reduction in the heart rate.

Stroke volume

The actual amount of blood ejected by a ventricle with each beat is dependent on the volume of blood entering the ventricle during diastole (end-diastolic volume, EDV) and the volume of blood left in the ventricle following systole (end-systolic volume, ESV) where stroke volume = EDV − ESV.

The EDV refers to the volume of blood entering a ventricle during diastole. This volume is determined principally by the length of time available for ventricular filling and the venous pressure (preload). The ventricles normally increase their volume to 120 ml.

The ESV refers to the volume of blood remaining in a ventricle following systole and is normally around 50 ml. The ESV is determined principally by arterial pressure or resistance to blood flow offered by the arterial system (afterload), and the force of ventricular contraction.

The force of ventricular contraction: Starling's law

The force of contraction of cardiac muscle is proportional to the resting length of the muscle fibres. Therefore, within physiological limits, the more the heart is filled with blood during diastole, the greater the degree to which the muscle fibres are stretched. This results in a greater force of contraction, increasing the volume of blood ejected from the ventricle with each contraction (stroke volume). This is the basis of Starling's law of the heart.

Nevertheless, the work achieved by the heart cannot increase indefinitely. A maximum is reached such that, although increased filling of the heart produces increased contraction over the normal range of volumes, beyond this point the heart becomes overdistended and less effective as a pump.

The property of the cardiac muscle described by Starling's law, in allowing stroke volume to be adjusted in response to the volume of blood returning to the heart (venous return), works in conjunction with the sympathetic nervous system to increase the stroke volume and decrease the ESV, thus ensuring that the volume of blood in the heart is kept within the range over which Starling's law operates most effectively.

SUMMARY

This chapter offers an introduction to the anatomy of the heart, the physiology involved in the cardiac cycle and the regulation of cardiac output. The principles outlined will serve as a necessary precursor to understanding the pathophysiology of dysrhythmias and heart disease, and also the nursing care required in the management of patients with cardiac problems.

FURTHER READING

Ashworth, P., Clarke, C. (eds.) (1992). *Cardiovascular Intensive Care Nursing*, Churchill Livingstone, Edinburgh.

Goodall, C.J. (1994). *Exploring Physiology: An Interactive Workbook for Nurses*. Unit 3 Circulatory Systems, Churchill Livingstone, Edinburgh, pp 77–118.

Hinchcliffe, S., Montague, S. (1988). Physiology for nursing practice, in *Cardiovascular Function*, Balliere Tindall, London, pp 315–394.

Rutishauser, S. (1994). *Physiology and Anatomy: A Basis for Nursing and Health Care*, Churchill Livingstone, Edinburgh, pp. 77–106.

Schamroth, L. (1982). *An Introduction to Electrocardiography* (6th edn), Blackwell Scientific Publications, Oxford.

Tortora, G.J., Anagnostakos, N.P. (1987). Principles of anatomy and physiology, in *The Cardiovascular System: Heart*, Harper and Row, New York, pp.461–486.

2.

ASSESSMENT OF THE CARDIAC PATIENT

An accurate assessment of the patient forms the foundation stone on which planning, implementation and evaluation of care is based. It is the baseline from which the nursing care is formulated and its effectiveness evaluated.

With current professional debate on the use of nursing models and the growing use of computerised patient care systems, there are many different formats on which the assessment information is based. Indeed it may be shaped and determined locally. In addition, each member of the health care team will take a different focus on assessment. However, in order to make an informed decision about care planning, the nurse must be able to use and integrate data from other disciplines. In this way, independent and interdependent nursing functions can be prioritised according to the needs of the patient.

Patients with cardiac disorders may become unstable over a very short period of time. Therefore it is essential that patient assessment is individualised and prioritised according to specific patient needs. The nurse must use her or his discretion as to what history and observations are crucial to care planning, which other sources are available so that the nurse can become more informed about the process of care for the cardiac patient.

COMPREHENSIVE NURSING ASSESSMENT

The following areas represent a spectrum of all the information that can be used in care planning; some information is central to the care, e.g. the nature of the problem presenting, while some is peripheral. Again, it rests with the individual nurse to select relevant details to be obtained in the assessment of that specific patient, at that specific time.

The nurse experienced in caring for patients with cardiac problems will be able to focus on and 'troubleshoot' potential patient problems. On receiving information that a patient is to be admitted, the expert nurse will draw from knowledge and experience to prioritise the care that the patient may require. However, this does not mean that all other areas have to be neglected or ignored; all aspects must receive some consideration in the assessment process. During the initial assessment, it is important to take a few minutes to validate all relevant patient biographic details (e.g. name, address, next of kin).

ASSESSING THE GENERAL APPEARANCE OF THE PATIENT

It is during the initial contact with the patient that useful information can be gained by taking a general impression of the following:

- Skin colour and warmth.
- Shortness of breath interfering with speech.
- Posture and movement in bed: Is the patient sitting forward suggesting pericarditis, sitting upright suggestive of cardiac failure, or agitated suggesting acute myocardial infarction?
- Distension of neck veins: Does the body move with each heart beat, are there bounding neck pulses, Corrigan's pulses, suggesting severe aortic regurgitation?
- Body weight: Is the patient undernourished or cachexic suggesting severe heart failure?
- Level of consciousness: Do thought processes reflect cerebral perfusion or low cardiac output?
- Level of distress or anxiety.

Taking a top-down approach, observations from looking at the face may indicate overt cardiac disorders, for example:

Facial characteristics:
- Malar flush suggesting rheumatic fever with mitral disorder.
- Café au lait complexion suggesting infective endocarditis.
- Jaundice suggesting hepatic engorgement.
- Facial oedema suggesting constrictive pericarditis or tricuspid valve disease.
- Diagonal earlobe crease (McCarthy's sign) may indicate coronary artery disease.

Colour:
- Peripheral cyanosis (e.g. on nose, lips, ear lobes) suggesting vasoconstriction from anxiety, cold or low-output state.
- Central cyanosis of buccal mucosa suggesting serious cardiac or pulmonary disease.
- Pallor suggesting anaemia or increased vasoconstriction.
- Jaundice due to hepatic engorgement from right ventricular failure.

Eyes:
- Corneal arcus (thin, grey–white circle around iris): if seen in young (not black) people it suggests hypercholesterolaemia.
- Xanthelasmas (rounded yellowish plaques nasal side of eyelids) may occur naturally, or may indicate hyperlipoproteinaemia.
- Petechial and subconjunctival haemorrhages suggesting of infective endocarditis.

This type of assessment data can be collected easily while watching and listening to the patient, e.g. when establishing the main reasons for hospital admission. This information sets the scene for further assessment questions and helps to prioritise care planning.

CARE PLANNING

Present problem

The main reason for seeking medical care is highlighted in the patient's perception. If an active problem exists, e.g. chest pain, further assessment should be limited to essential information to alleviate the problem. In this instance, it may also be more appropriate to modify the use of open questions and to use of 'yes/no' answers. It should always borne in mind that if a patient is known/susceptible to cardiac disease, any pain should be considered to be secondary to ischaemia until proven otherwise. Equally there is no correlation between the degree of chest pain and the seriousness of the problem and any pain the patient may be experiencing can be referred cardiac pain, e.g. to the jaw or fingers.

Present illness

This allows further discussion and exploration of the duration of the problem with any associated signs and symptoms. The nature, intensity, location and radiation of any previous pain should be noted, together with any exacerbating or relieving factors.

Past medical history

Further information is discussed in order to develop a broader picture of the patient. Information regarding past illnesses, hospital admissions, medications and allergies is elicited. This may reveal evidence to support the original patient problem or give pointers as to potential concerns.

Family history

Again this enriches the picture that is being built up of the patient, not only in terms of medical disease but also regarding family exposure and coping with hospital and illness. Any incidence of cardiac disease or medical problems (particularly hypertension, diabetes mellitus or hyperlipidaemia) within the family is noted and relevant areas can be explored. Having determined the major issues, if appropriate, a more global assessment can now continue and the format followed will be directed by the model in use.

Areas that should involve some discussion encompass a more detailed picture of the patient's perception of the problem, together with an understanding of the patient's and family's normal coping mechanisms and the resources and support (in terms of personal social and economic sources) available. It is sometimes difficult to establish realistic indicators of the patient's perception of illness, one method is to establish what activities the patient envisages performing in, for example, 4 weeks' time and what lifestyle changes he or she would be prepared to make if this could not be achieved. In respect of privacy to the patient, these are not always areas one can engage in within a few minutes of meeting. It may be more appropriate to follow up further discussions on this after a deeper trust is established.

CARDIOVASCULAR ASSESSMENT SKILLS

During the assessment process for the patient with a cardiac disorder, some assessments have a greater significance. These areas are now explored.

Arterial pulse

This can yield information as to the efficiency of the heart as a pump. A normal pulse contour has a smooth and rapid upstroke. However, a small, weak pulse usually indicates a reduced stroke volume and ejection fraction, and/or increased vasoconstriction (systemic vascular resistance). Irregular rhythms, e.g. ventricular ectopics, can be identified by an occasional irregular pulse, or atrial fibrillation by an 'irregularly irregular' pulse.

The radial pulse should always be used for assessment unless the patient is shocked or in cardiac arrest. Patients with tachycardia should have apex and radial pulse rates recorded during the same minute. The rationale for this is that as the heart rate increases the diastolic and therefore ventricular filling time shortens. This is reflected in a reduced stroke volume and therefore possible absent peripheral pulses.

Blood pressure

The blood pressure (BP) is an indicator of the cardiac output. Therefore any patient receiving vasoactive drugs (e.g. dobutamine) will need close and frequent BP recordings. If frequent BP readings are required, noninvasive BP monitoring (e.g. using Dinamapp) can be used, which is less disturbing to the patient.

When taking an accurate BP reading it is important that the correct size cuff for the circumference of the arm is used, e.g. the bladder width should be 40% of the circumference of the patient's arm at the mid point. Any irregular rhythm will make accurate BP measurement difficult because of inadequate ventricular filling and stroke volume. Patients with a dissecting aortic aneurysm or with occlusive arterial disease will have unequal BP in both arms. In the obese patient, a standard adult cuff can be applied to the forearm 13 cm from the elbow and the radial pulse used to auscultate. To take thigh readings, e.g. to check for dissecting aortic aneurysm or coarctation of the aorta, apply the cuff over the mid thigh and auscultate at the popliteal artery.

The use of standing/lying cuff readings reflects postural hypotension, which in cardiac patients is most commonly caused by a fluid deficit secondary to saline depletion, inadequate vasoconstrictor mechanisms, or autonomic insufficiency.

The normal reaction to lying down and then standing up is to increase the heart rate by 15% and to drop the systolic and diastolic pressure by 10–15 mmHg. This fact is therefore important when caring for those on antihypertensive agents, vasodilators or calcium-channel blockers.

The pulse pressure, i.e. the difference between systolic and diastolic pressures, reflects stroke volume, ejection strength and systemic vascular resistance. It indicates loosely the body's ability to maintain cardiac output. Its significance can be seen in a widened pulse pressure as seen in bradycardia, complete heart block, aortic regurgitation, anxiety and exercise. In contrast, a narrowed pulse pressure can be seen in heart failure, shock, hypovolaemia, mechanical obstruction in aortic stenosis, mitral stenosis and peripheral vasoconstriction.

Paradoxical blood pressure is the exaggerated decrease (10 mmHg or greater) in systolic pressure during inspiration. Its significance during assessment is that it occurs diagnostically in cardiac tamponade, also in chronic airway disease, pulmonary embolism and restrictive cardiomyopathy.

Jugular venous/central venous pressure

Jugular venous pressure (JVP) reflects the pressures in the right side of the heart but is not necessarily a true reflection of events in the left side. The JVP is usually 'read' from the internal jugular vein with the patient sitting up at 45° angle. In health, this vein is not normally visible but, in illness the JVP can be measured as the distance above the sternal angle (in cm). The normal value is 4–10 cm above the level of the right atrium.

The JVP waveform reflects events occurring within the heart and can be labelled a, c and v waves and x and y descents. It is through identification of abnormalities in these that primary cardiac disturbances can be identified. For example, the a wave represents the small amount of blood that flows back into the superior vena cava during atrial contraction. In atrial dysrhythmias, e.g. atrial fibrillation, this will not occur because there is no organised atrial activity and therefore the a wave is absent. Conversely, canon (giant) a waves are seen in atrioventricular dissociation, when the right atrium contracts against a closed tricuspid valve.

The central venous pressure is now monitored frequently in the clinical setting. It is important to establish right atrial pressures and to determine the effectiveness of fluid and drug management. Intravenous access is obtained through the subclavian, jugular, brachial or femoral approach. Intermittent readings (in cmH$_2$0) are taken using a manometer or continuously with a monitor (in mmHg). The normal recording is 4–10 cm (above water); 1 mmHg being equivalent to 1.36 cmH$_2$0. Readings above 10 cm indicate right ventricular failure, late left ventricular failure, hypervolaemia, or superior vena cava obstruction, while readings below normal may indicate hypovolaemia.

Heart

The assessment of the heart, at present performed when assessing the medical history, consists of processes of inspection, palpation, percussion and auscultation.

Inspection involves identifying any abnormal impulses referred through the chest wall as abnormal pulsating movements, as in aortic aneurysm or ventricular enlargement. Hand palpation may reveal thrills or pulsations indicative of aneurysm or valvular dysfunction. During percussion, the size of the heart is evaluated by ascertaining whether the underlying structures are solid or air- or fluid-filled. Lastly, auscultation will reveal any cardiac murmurs caused by turbulent blood flow.

Briefly, the normal heart beat consists of the first (closure of the mitral and tricuspid valves – the lubb) and second (closure of aortic and pulmonary valves – the dupp) sound. Other heart sounds such as S3, S4, pericardial friction rubs, splits, opening snaps, ejection clicks and murmurs, may warn of abnormal flow and turbulence within the heart or great vessels.

Venous circulation

Oedema is the abnormal accumulation of fluid in the interstitial spaces. It is caused by right-sided failure, hypoalbuminaemia and excessive renal retention of sodium and water. Bilateral oedema suggests a systemic aetiology, while unilateral oedema may be a more local problem. It is important to remember that a weight gain of 10 pounds or an increase of 5 litres of extracellular fluid volume can precede visible oedema. Interstitial oedema is dependent on position. Pitting oedema is seen if after a 5-second pressure there is a depression mark left on the skin. In long-standing oedema, there may be pigmentation or reddening of the skin in the lower extremities.

Skin extremities

These observations can be carried out unobtrusively through the nurse's appropriate use of touch. Arm-to-arm and leg-to-leg comparisons should be made; note should also be made if cool and moist (stress response) or cold and clammy (shocked state). A sluggish capillary refill time, seen by depressing and then releasing the tip of the fingernail, is suggestive of slower capillary flow, as in heart failure. Clubbing of the fingernails is associated with chronic haemoglobin desaturation and congenital heart disease; its aetiology is unknown. The diagnosis is made by the presence of 180° or greater angle between the base of the nail and skin next to the cuticle. In addition, Osler's nodes (tender erythematous lesions on the hands and feet) are indicative of infective endocarditis.

Cardiovascular assessment would not be complete without the inclusion of ECG observation. It is not within the remit of this chapter to cover this aspect in detail, except to say that valuable data can be gained from observation of cardiac monitors and 12-lead ECGs to augment the nursing assessment data already obtained. In addition to recognising the obvious life-threatening dysrhythmias, particular emphasis should be placed on recognising infarction patterns, ischaemic episodes or areas, developing heart block and increasing irritability within the conduction system (ectopic activity).

Body temperature

A few quick reminders about this aspect of assessment follow. Many patients who have sustained a myocardial infarction will have a low-grade pyrexia as a result of a nonspecific response to myocardial necrosis. In addition, those with pericarditis will also exhibit a low-grade pyrexia caused by the inflammatory response. Patients who are tachypnoeic or receiving oxygen will record lower oral temperatures because of a cooling effect and, if an axilla temperature is recorded using a standard mercury thermometer, it must remain *in situ* for at least 9 minutes for accuracy.

Lungs

As stated previously, the nurse can obtain information regarding the respiratory status of the patient purely by watching and listening. In addition, similar principles can be used as in cardiac assessment.

Inspection will reveal the:

* Respiratory rate, depth and rhythm. Tachypnoea may be associated with cardiac failure, bradypnoea in those who may be depressed cerebrally or may have had recent administration of opiates, while Cheynes–Stokes respiration may be associated with severe left ventricular failure.
* Presence of a cough or any sputum. A dry, hacking cough is common in pulmonary congestion from cardiac failure, while pink frothy sputum is indicative of pulmonary oedema.
* Ease of respiration. Use of accessory muscles indicates respiratory difficulty, while guarding indicates pain.
* Chest configuration. A barrel chest is associated with emphysema, while spinal abnormalities may hinder chest expansion.

Palpation and percussion will confirm the presence of any fluid or solid tissue replacing air-filled spaces; this can then be confirmed further by auscultation. By listening to the anterior and posterior aspects of the thorax, the presence of crackles (fluid in the alveoli or the explosive reopening of alveoli sounding similar to rubbing several strands of hair between thumb and forefinger in front of the ear) from heart failure, atelectasis and wheezes (rapid air movement through constricted airways revealed by the production of musical sounds of varying pitch, usually during expiration) from obstructive lung disease or compression of small airways through interstitial oedema will be heard.

CONCLUSION

The areas covered in this chapter give a focused view on cardiac assessment skills. As already stated, the purpose of assessment is to give purpose and direction to care – it establishes a baseline. It is important that, when making future assessments on the patient, trends are identified and acted on. Any abnormal readings must be reported so that further planning, implementation and evaluation of care can occur. Throughout this process, the patient must remain the central focus of care. The relationship established by the nurse with the patient and close family and friends allows for the sharing of information. This facilitates informed decision-making and an active participation in care, which is a prerequisite if the cardiac patient is to learn to manage successfully their cardiac disorder.

Patient assessment: key features

These may be summarised as follows:

- Accurate and timely assessment forms the foundation stone for the process of care.
- Assessment must be individualised and prioritised according to patient needs.
- Trend is more important than individual readings.
- Observations are only of use if the nurse understands their importance and significance.
- To make an informed decision about care planning, the nurse must be able to use and integrate data from all disciplines.

FURTHER READING

Guzzetta, C.E. Siefert, P.C. (1991). Cardiovascular assessment, in *Comprehensive Cardiac Care* (7th edn.) Kinney, M. R., Packa, D. R., Andreoli, K. G. and Zipes, D. P. (eds), Mosby Year Book, St Louis.
Nurse Review (1987). *Cardiac Problems,* Springhouse, USA.
Thompson, D., Webster, R. (1992). *Caring for the Coronary Patient,* Butterworth-Heinemann, Oxford.
Underhill, S. L., Woods, S.L., Froelicher, E.S.S. Halpenny, C.J. (1989). *Cardiac Nursing (*2nd edn.), J. B. Lippincott, Philadelphia.

3.

CARDIAC PHARMACOLOGY

This chapter provides essential information about some of the drugs commonly used in the treatment of patients suffering from ischaemic heart disease and myocardial infarction. Detailed information, including standard dosages, should be obtained from the manufacturer's literature, the current *British National Formulary*, or by consultation with a pharmacist. Owing to rapid advances in medical pharmacology, new drugs are being introduced frequently in this field, so groups of drugs with examples, rather than specific drugs, are often referred to. The following drugs, or groups of drugs, are included:

- Analgesics.
- Antiarrhythmics.
- Angiotensin converting enzyme inhibitors.
- Anticoagulants.
- Beta blockers.

- Digoxin.
- Diuretics.
- Inotropes.
- Nitrates.
- Magnesium.

DRUGS USED DURING CARDIAC EMERGENCIES

Oxygen

During cardiac emergencies, cardiac output is severely reduced or absent. Tissue hypoxia develops rapidly in the absence of effective circulation; however, the administration of oxygen may reduce this effect. Oxygen should be administered in the highest concentration available. Patients with long-standing hypercapnia (usually those with chronic pulmonary disease) still require high concentrations of oxygen, despite concerns for their respiratory drive. When cardiac output is absent, reoxygenation is the immediate priority. Respiratory arrest will follow cardiac arrest so the patient's ventilation will inevitably require support.

Large quantities of oxygen may be required during an emergency and the provision of adequate supplies is essential. Oxygen from a piped, central supply is clearly unlimited; oxygen cylinders, in contrast, are emptied quickly and back-up supplies must be organised before supplies are exhausted.

Adrenaline

Adrenaline is a naturally occurring stimulant. It is a hormone, produced in the medulla of the adrenal glands, that acts on both alpha and beta sympathetic receptors within the body organs.

Effects

Adrenaline:

- Acts as a positive inotrope by increasing the force and rate of ventricular concentration.
- Causes peripheral vasoconstriction, without constriction of the cerebral or coronary vessels, thereby improving cerebral and myocardial circulation.
- Relaxes smooth muscle, including the bronchial tree, thereby increasing airway diameter.
- Raises blood sugar levels by mobilising glucose stores.

Adrenaline cannot be administered orally since it is destroyed by stomach acid. In emergencies, it may be given intravenously or endobronchially (via an endotracheal tube), where it is rapidly absorbed through the respiratory mucosa. In the past, adrenaline was administered via intracardiac injection directly into the left ventricle; however, this route of administration is hazardous and may result in serious complications, such as coronary artery rupture, and is therefore no longer recommended.

Indications

Adrenaline is used during cardiac arrest to provoke ventricular fibrillation in an asystolic heart. Defibrillation can then be attempted. In 'fine' or low-amplitude ventricular fibrillation, adrenaline may be given to produce 'coarse' or high-amplitude ventricular fibrillation, a rhythm that is more susceptible to defibrillation. It is also thought that adrenaline administered during cardiac arrest may reduce or prevent cerebral damage, since its vasoconstrictive effects redirect blood flow from the stomach and nonessential tissues, to vital organs such as the brain and the heart. Occasionally, adrenaline is used in an intravenous infusion as inotropic support.

Notes

Adrenaline causes pupillary dilatation and therefore, once it has been administered, pupil reactions must not be used as an indication of cerebral function. Adrenaline is inactivated if mixed with sodium bicarbonate solution. If only one point of venous access is available, careful flushing of the cannula before and after the injection of adrenaline is essential. Preferably, a separate infusion point should be used for bicarbonate, if required. Monitoring of blood sugar level may be required if an adrenaline infusion is used, or in patients with abnormal glucose tolerance, e.g. in diabetes mellitus.

Atropine

Atropine is an anticholinergic drug, i.e. it blocks the action of acetylcholine at the parasympathetic nerve endings. It has many actions, including the blocking of the actions of the vagus nerve on the SA node. Vagal activity slows the heart rate, so blocking its activity will therefore increase the heart rate. It is given either intravenously or endobronchially.

Indications
Atropine is used in the treatment of bradycardia, when cardiac output is compromised. It is effective in the treatment of bradycardia resulting from excessive vagal action but is not always effective when bradycardia results from other causes (e.g. AV conduction defects). Atropine is also used in conjunction with adrenaline in the treatment of asystole, in order to provoke ventricular activity.

Notes
Atropine causes dilatation of the pupil and also paralysis of the muscles of the eye that affect accommodation, resulting in blurring of near vision. Urinary retention may be a problem, especially in the elderly.

Calcium

Calcium ions are critical for normal myocardial conduction and contraction, indeed, calcium ions in the form of calcium gluconate or calcium chloride may be used during cardiac arrest. Increasing the extracellular/intracellular calcium gradient (by injecting calcium into the blood) promotes an increase in the concentration of calcium ions within the cells. Calcium is particularly helpful in hyperkalaemia, in stabilising cell membranes, and protecting against dysrhythmias.

Indications
Calcium is indicated in the treatment of loss of cardiac output caused by electromechanical dissociation, also when calcium antagonist toxicity is suspected (i.e. toxic blood levels of drugs such as verapamil). It may also be used in life-threatening dysrhythmias caused by hyperkalaemia, or if hypocalcaemia exists.

Notes
Calcium must not be mixed with sodium bicarbonate solution since precipitation will occur. Calcium cannot be given endobronchially.

Lignocaine

Lignocaine is an antiarrhythmic agent used in the treatment of ventricular dysrhythmias. It reduces myocardial excitability, with only a slight negative inotropic effect. Nevertheless, it should be avoided if possible in patients with low cardiac output. Lignocaine is given intravenously since it is rapidly metabolised by the liver. The effects are short-lived, lasting approximately 20 minutes; thus a loading dose is usually followed by an infusion, which is gradually reduced over a period of hours as the dysrhythmia resolves.

Indications
Lignocaine is used in ventricular tachycardia. It may also be used if multiple ventricular ectopics are compromising cardiac output, or if 'R on T' ectopic activity may provoke ventricular fibrillation. Lignocaine may also be used after an episode of ventricular fibrillation to prevent recurrence.

Notes

Neurological side-effects such as restlessness, confusion and convulsions can occur. Significant plasma levels may be achieved by subcutaneous infiltration for use during certain procedures, e.g. during pacemaker insertion. Lignocaine is less effective if hypokalaemia exists and is not indicated in the treatment of supraventricular dysrhythmias.

Sodium bicarbonate solution

Sodium bicarbonate solution is given to correct the metabolic acidosis that may develop during cardiac arrest. It is only required if significant acidosis has been established by arterial pH measurement or, in the absence of such a measurement, if resuscitation is prolonged. Small amounts are administered by bolus injection (or occasionally by carefully controlled infusion).

Indications

Significant metabolic acidosis caused by cardiac arrest.

Notes

Sodium bicarbonate solution must not be mixed with other drugs, especially adrenaline and calcium, since inactivation or precipitation may occur. A separate infusion line, preferably a central line, should be used; however, this may not be possible in an emergency situation.

Analgesics

Opiate analgesia is often required to relieve the pain associated with acute myocardial infarction, diamorphine or morphine being the drugs of choice. Given intravenously opiates are rapidly effective, and the dosage should be repeated to ensure that the patient is kept pain-free. Intramuscular injection should be avoided since it is painful and absorption may be unpredictable if the patient is peripherally vasoconstricted. Intramuscular injections are also contraindicated following thrombolytic therapy and they may alter the serum enzyme profile.

Effects

As well as powerful analgesic effects, diamorphine reduces anxiety, which is obviously beneficial in acute myocardial infarction. Haemodynamic effects (probably vasodilatation, although the exact mechanism is unknown) will reduce pulmonary oedema, if present.

Indications

Analgesics are used for chest pain associated with acute myocardial infarction. Opiates are also useful in acute left ventricular failure because of the anxiolytic and haemodynamic effects.

Notes

Pain results in an increase in endogenous adrenaline secretion which may precipitate dysrhythmias following myocardial infarction. Thus adequate analgesia is crucial, both in terms of patient comfort and in the prevention of complications. Opiates (when administered initially) and myocardial infarction both cause nausea and vomiting. Apart from the distress caused to the patient, vomiting increases cardiac workload and may worsen ischaemia. The changes in intrathoracic pressure that occur during vomiting can lead to vagal stimulation and may precipitate bradydysrhythmias. It is important, therefore, that prophylactic anti-emetics are given initially with opiate analgesia (the emetic effects of opiates reduce gradually after repeated administration).

Sedation will occur when opiates are administered, and close observation of respiratory effort is required since hypoxia must be avoided. Oxygen therapy may be required and, if respiratory depression is life-threatening, an opiate antagonist (such as naloxone) may be used to reverse respiratory depression. Naloxone is rapidly effective but relatively short-lived; repeated doses may therefore be required.

Constipation is an almost inevitable result of opiate administration and, while not of immediate significance, should be considered, because straining at stool can also precipitate bradydysrhythmias. Prophylactic laxatives may be indicated, especially when high fluid and fibre intake are contraindicated.

Antiarrhythmic drugs

All antiarrhythmics, with the exception of digoxin, are cardiac depressants and therefore have a negative inotropic effect. This effect is more marked with some drugs than others, such that disopyramide, quinidine, flecainide are most negatively inotropic, beta blockers are next, while verapamil, lignocaine and amiodarone are least negatively inotropic. Any patient receiving antiarrhythmic medication should be observed closely, to detect any adverse effect on cardiac output. Whenever possible, such drugs should be avoided in patients with cardiac failure, unless the failure is caused by the arrhythmia. Particular care must be taken if a patient is receiving more than one of these drugs, since interactions may exacerbate depressant effects, e.g. beta blockers combined with verapamil may result in asystole.

Classification

A classification of antiarrhythmic drugs was proposed by Vaughan Williams in 1970, according to the mode of action of the drugs. Four classes have been identified.

Class 1: Includes drugs with membrane-stabilising activities. The class has been subdivided according to the effects of the drug on the cells in the bundle of His.

Class 1A	Class 1B	Class 1C
Quinidine.	Lignocaine.	Flecainide.
Procainamide.	Tocainide.	
Disopyramide.	Mexiletine.	

Class 2: Includes drugs with antiadrenergic activities, i.e. beta blockers. By blocking beta-adrenergic receptors in the heart, the stimulatory effects of endogenous adrenaline are reduced. Beta blockers are now more commonly used in the treatment of hypertension and angina.

Class 3: This group includes drugs that prolong the refractory period of atrial and ventricular muscle (i.e. the period when the myocardium will not respond to stimulation), e.g. amiodarone.

Class 4: This group includes drugs that interfere with the flow of calcium ions into muscle cells of arterial walls, leading to relaxation of the muscle and consequent vasodilatation. The result is a lowering of the blood pressure, and improved coronary perfusion. (e.g. nifedipine, diltiazem, nicardipine). These drugs can therefore be used in the treatment of angina and hypertension. In addition, some of the drugs in this category, notably verapamil, affect myocardial cells thus reducing the force of ventricular contraction and slowing conduction, and so can be used in the treatment of tachydysrhythmias.

Amiodarone

Effects
Amiodarone has only a minimal negative effect on cardiac output. It also has the advantage that it can be given either intravenously or orally. Owing to its long half-life, a loading dose of amiodarone is required, followed by a lower maintenance dose once therapeutic plasma levels have been achieved. It is important that the patient understands this reduction in dose in order to comply accurately with the regime of medication once discharged.

Indications
Amiodarone is effective against both ventricular and supraventricular arrhythmias. It is also used in the treatment of re-entry tachycardias due to the presence of accessory conductive pathways, e.g. in the Wolff–Parkinson–White syndrome.

Notes
Bolus intravenous doses of amiodarone must be given slowly, since rapid injection results in profound hypotension. Peripheral infusion causes venous irritation: central lines should be used whenever possible. Side-effects are common and some are serious (e.g. pulmonary fibrosis) and may limit the therapeutic use of the drug. Photosensitivity occurs and patients must be warned to avoid sunbathing and to use sunblocks. Some patients complain of a metallic taste in the mouth.

Amiodarone contains iodine and may disrupt thyroid function. Regular thyroid function tests are required while amiodarone therapy is in progress.

Verapamil

Indications
Verapamil is particularly useful in the treatment of tachycardias that are supraventricular in origin. It is not indicated in ventricular tachycardia.

Notes
Verapamil can be given intravenously in emergencies, or orally as a maintenance therapy. Verapamil should be avoided if beta blockers have been given to the patient within 24 hours, since the cumulative effects can cause cardiac arrest.

Digoxin

The effects of digoxin are seen in the failing heart, most especially when atrial fibrillation is present. The value of digoxin as a cardiac stimulant in sinus rhythm is uncertain. Digoxin is the only antiarrhythmic agent in common use that has a positive effect on the cardiac output.

Effects
Digoxin increases the force of ventricular contraction by increasing the amount of intracellular calcium in the myocardium. The heart rate is slowed, owing to direct action on the SA node and by an increase in the activity of the vagus nerve. Conduction at the AV node, and in the bundle of His is depressed. These effects combine to increase the cardiac output, especially when the ventricular rate in atrial fibrillation is reduced.

Indications
Digoxin is used in the treatment of cardiac failure, particularly when the failure is caused or complicated by atrial fibrillation.

Notes
Digoxin may be given orally, intramuscularly or intravenously. A loading dose may be given where rapid action is required. Care must be taken in the administration of digoxin since confusion can arise when dosages are written in milligrams, as opposed to micrograms.

The pulse deficit of patients in atrial fibrillation should be monitored, by means of apex/radial recordings. The pulse deficit will fall as effective therapy is instituted.

Digoxin toxicity can cause serious arrhythmias and should be detected early. Toxicity is more likely in patients with impaired renal function, and in patients with hypokalaemia (which may occur as a result of diuretic therapy). Plasma digoxin levels should be measured to monitor treatment; however, general observation may reveal signs of developing toxicity. These include bradycardia (perhaps associated with 'coupling' when normal beats are followed by ventricular ectopics to produce a double pulsation), anorexia, nausea and vomiting and altered colour vision. ECG changes will also occur.

When bradycardia is detected, digoxin should be omitted. The dosage may require adjustment. A pulse rate of 60 beats/minute is usually regarded as the lowest acceptable rate. However, it is important that the apex rate is recorded in such a situation, since a radial rate below 60 beats/minute may be a reflection of a large pulse deficit.

Patients are not usually required to monitor their pulse following discharge since stabilisation of the digoxin therapy should have been achieved. They should, however, be aware of the signs of toxicity and have been instructed to consult a doctor should such signs occur.

Severe digoxin toxicity can be treated with an infusion of digoxin antibodies, which rapidly reverse the toxic effects, although this treatment is very expensive. During the administration of the antibodies, the patient must be observed for signs of hypersensitivity and anaphylaxis, since the antibodies are prepared from sheep protein.

Digoxin is not absorbed properly in the presence of antacids, so concurrent administration must be avoided, the digoxin and antacids being administered at least 1–2 hours apart. Caution is indicated when digitalised patients require cardioversion, since intractable dysrhythmias may result. It may be necessary to omit the digoxin therapy prior to the procedure.

Beta blockers

Beta blockers block the effects of adrenaline and noradrenaline on beta-adrenergic receptors in the sympathetic nervous system. Beta$_1$ receptors are located in the heart, while beta$_2$ receptors are found in the bronchi and in blood vessels. Some beta blockers are effective against both beta$_1$ and beta$_2$ receptors and are termed nonselective, e.g. propranolol, oxprenolol, timolol. Others have a greater effect on beta$_1$ receptors and are termed selective, e.g. atenolol, metoprolol, bisoprolol.

Effects
Beta blockers cause a reduction in heart rate and cardiac workload. Myocardial excitability is decreased, cardiac output is lowered and cardiac failure may be precipitated. Blood pressure is also reduced. Nonselective beta blockers (i.e. those effective against both beta$_1$ and beta$_2$ receptors) cause bronchospasm and may cause problems in asthmatic patients. Peripheral vasoconstriction will also occur. Central nervous system effects may cause vivid dreams or nightmares. Symptoms of anxiety such as palpitations, tremor and sweating are also relieved, so beta blockers may be used to control these symptoms.

Indications
Beta blockers are used in the treatment of angina, hypertension and cardiac arrhythmias. Recent evidence suggests that the administration of beta blockers following myocardial infarction may reduce the incidence of myocardial rupture.

Notes
Beta blockers should be used with caution in patients suffering from asthma and peripheral vascular disease since these conditions may be exacerbated. Caution is also required in the treatment of diabetic patients as the symptoms of hypoglycaemia are masked. Beta blockers are negative inotropes and must be avoided in patients with cardiac failure, or those likely to suffer cardiac failure, including patients immediately following acute myocardial infarction.

Diuretics

Diuretics increase the amount of urine excreted via the kidney, by decreasing the amount of water and electrolytes reabsorbed in the renal tubules. They are classified according to their site of action in the renal tubule. Thiazide diuretics such as bendrofluazide and loop diuretics such as frusemide, cause potassium depletion and supplementation may be required. Potassium-sparing diuretics, such as amiloride and spironolactone, can be used but are less effective at causing fluid loss. Thus a combination of types of diuretic is often used.

Effects
Increased urine output reduces the circulating blood volume and so reduces preload, i.e. the amount of blood returning to the heart in the venous system. This in turn reduces cardiac workload. Peripheral and pulmonary oedema are reduced.

Indications
Diuretics are indicated in acute and chronic cardiac failure. They may also contribute to the treatment of hypertension.

Notes
Intravenous frusemide is the drug of choice in the treatment of acute left-ventricular failure. Administered via this route, an almost immediate effect is seen and the diuresis is usually complete within 2 hours. The major side-effect of thiazide and loop diuretics, hypokalaemia, is particularly significant in the treatment of patients with cardiac disease. Hypokalaemia causes potentially life-threatening ventricular arrhythmias, including ventricular fibrillation. An increase in the frequency of ventricular ectopic activity may occur as an early sign. Patients receiving diuretic therapy require regular monitoring of serum potassium levels and supplementation prescribed as appropriate. Potassium supplements may be given orally or by intravenous infusion. Intravenous potassium must be diluted adequately prior to administration. Indiscriminate supplementation, that is, in the absence of blood results, is inadvisable since hyperkalaemia is equally dangerous. Hypokalaemia also potentiates digoxin toxicity and the combination of digoxin and diuretic therapy is common in the treatment of cardiac failure.

Acutely ill patients receiving diuretic therapy require an accurate assessment of fluid balance and, when possible, the patient should be weighed daily, as this can be a more accurate measure of fluid balance than fluid balance charts. Blood pressure must also monitored, since a large diuresis may result in hypovolaemia, causing blood pressure to fall. A postural drop in systolic blood pressure can often be detected in the early stages of hypovolaemia, thus recording lying and standing blood pressures may provide an early indication of dehydration.

ACE inhibitors

Angiotensin converting enzyme (ACE) inhibitors (e.g. captopril, enalapril, lisinopril) interfere with the renin–angiotensin pathway, which constitutes part of the normal mechanism of blood-pressure control (Fig. 3-1). Renin is an enzyme produced in the kidney in response to reduced blood pressure. The reduced renal blood flow is detected in the juxtaglomerular apparatus in the renal arteriole, which then secretes renin into the bloodstream. Renin then converts angiotensinogen into angiotensin I, which is then converted into an active hormone, angiotensin

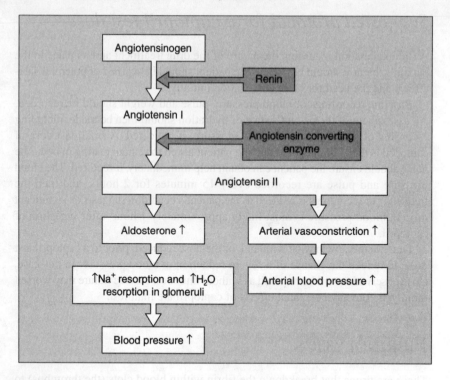

Fig. 3-1 Diagram of the renin–angiotensin pathway.

II, in the lungs, in the presence of angiotensin converting enzyme. Angiotensin II causes vasoconstriction and an increase in aldosterone secretion from the adrenal cortex, leading to sodium and water retention by the kidneys. Both of these actions raise the blood pressure.

Effects

Angiotensin converting enzyme inhibitors prevent the formation of angiotensin II, so the vasoconstriction and increase in blood volume caused by increased aldosterone production do not occur, thus reducing the blood pressure.

Indications

ACE inhibitors are used in the treatment of cardiac failure by reducing circulatory volume and cardiac afterload. They can also be used to treat hypertension.

Notes

ACE inhibitors can cause a profound drop in blood pressure, especially when the treatment is first introduced. This is more likely to occur if the patient is receiving diuretic therapy, particularly if the patient is hypovolaemic. For this reason, patients are often admitted to hospital for observation as the drugs are introduced. Therapy is often commenced with a test dose of captopril, which is relatively rapid in onset and short-acting. Once stabilised on captopril, a longer-acting ACE inhibitor such as enalapril can be used, since these drugs can be given as a once-daily dose.

Suggested protocol for a captopril test dose

A full explanation regarding the nature of the drug treatment and its place in the patient's therapy should be given. The patient should be warned of potential side-effects and the need for close observation initially.

Baseline recordings of blood pressure, pulse and weight should be recorded. An assessment of the patient's state of hydration should then be made, including recording of postural drop in blood pressure, if indicated. A small test dose of captopril is then administered and the patient asked to remain resting in bed. The nurse should ensure the patient can obtain help immediately, if required. The blood pressure and pulse are recorded every 15 minutes for 2 hours, and then the frequency of recordings is reduced as the patient's condition suggests. A significant drop in blood pressure is most likely approximately 1 hour after ingestion of captopril.

Diuretic therapy may be withheld, or the dose reduced, prior to a captopril test dose, to reduce the chance of a severe reduction in blood pressure. In this case, close observation will be required as without diuretics, cardiac failure may worsen rapidly, before any beneficial effects of captopril are manifest.

FIBRINOLYTICS

These are drugs that breakdown the fibrin within blood clots (the thrombus) to restore normal circulation. They are used following myocardial infarction to restore circulation to the damaged myocardium by unblocking occluded coronary arteries. Two categories are in use: nonspecific thrombolytic agents and fibrin-specific thrombolytic agents.

Fibrin-specific thrombolytic agents, such as anisoylated plasminogen streptokinase activator (APSAC) and recombinant tissue-plasminogen activator (rtPA), carry less risk of systemic side-effects, notably haemorrhage, because their actions are largely confined to the site of the thrombus; nevertheless, both drugs are expensive.

Streptokinase is a nonspecific thrombolytic agent and is the drug of choice in the treatment of myocardial infarction. Fibrin-specific agents are reserved for situations when the use of streptokinase would be inappropriate.

Streptokinase

Streptokinase must be given as quickly as possible once the diagnosis of myocardial infarction has been established. Most effective re-perfusion is achieved if treatment is given within 4 hours of the onset of symptoms; however, some benefits may result from treatment initiated within the first 12 hours.

Streptokinase causes systemic disruption to blood-clotting processes, haemorrhage is therefore a risk. Patients with a pre-existing risk of haemorrhage, including patients with a history of cerebrovascular disease, gastrointestinal haemorrhage, recent surgery or trauma, severe hypertension, liver disease and during pregnancy, must not be treated with streptokinase. Patients who have received streptokinase must not be injected intramuscularly.

Streptokinase is an exotoxin produced by streptococcal bacteria. It is therefore antigenic and so allergic reactions to streptokinase can occur. Administration of intravenous chlorpheniramine and hydrocortisone will reduce the allergic response. Patients who have had a recent streptococcal infection (often manifested as a sore throat) or who have received a previous dose of streptokinase within 6 months to 1 year are more likely to suffer an allergic reaction, so a fibrin-specific thrombolytic agent, e.g. recombinant tissue-plasminogen activator, should be used.

Streptokinase is administered by intravenous infusion over 1 hour, during which close observation of the patient should be maintained because, in addition to allergic reactions, reperfusion dysrhythmias may occur, since toxic metabolites are washed out of the ischaemic tissues as the circulation is restored.

ANTICOAGULANTS

A variety of anticoagulant drugs, including heparin, warfarin and aspirin, have been used in conjunction with fibrinolytic agents in an attempt to reduce the risk of thrombus reoccurrence following myocardial infarction. Research continues but results to date suggest that low-dose aspirin therapy may be the most appropriate choice.

Aspirin

Low-dose aspirin inhibits prostaglandin synthesis in platelets, which reduces platelet adhesiveness. Aspirin has also been used in unstable angina in an attempt to reduce the incidence of myocardial infarction. Following myocardial infarction, aspirin may reduce the recurrence of thrombus formation, particularly if used in conjunction with fibrinolytic therapy.

Aspirin is given orally, although the optimal therapeutic dose has not yet been established. Some patients for whom fibrinolytic therapy is contraindicated can receive aspirin safely, although some contraindications apply to both treatments.

Heparin

Heparin may be given subcutaneously to patients on bed rest following myocardial infarction, to reduce the incidence of deep vein thrombosis.

POSITIVE INOTROPES

Positive inotropes are drugs that increase the force of ventricular contraction, thereby improving the cardiac output. Examples include dopamine, dobutamine, adrenaline and isoprenaline. These drugs are used in the treatment of cardiogenic shock ('pump' failure) following myocardial infarction, to improve blood pressure and maintain perfusion of vital organs. Dopamine and dobutamine are most commonly used.

Dopamine

Effects
Dopamine is a naturally occurring neurotransmitter that is converted to adrenaline in the body. It acts as a $beta_1$-receptor stimulant and causes an increase in the force of ventricular contraction and also dilatation of the renal arteries, thus increasing renal blood flow and reducing the risk of acute tubular necrosis.

Notes
Dopamine is administered by continuous infusion and should be given via a central venous line, since peripheral administration may lead to vasoconstriction and necrosis. If dopamine escapes into peripheral tissues, the use of phentolamine injected locally as an antidote may prevent necrosis. Dosage is calculated according to body weight and titrated according to the response in blood pressure. Lower doses of dopamine have an effect only on renal perfusion, the so-called 'renal dose'.

Cardiac effects become apparent in moderate dosage but increases in blood pressure may be accompanied by tachycardia. Higher doses may precipitate tachydysrhythmias and limit the amount of dopamine that can be administered safely.

Patients receiving dopamine therapy require constant observation and monitoring of blood pressure, pulse, cardiac rhythm and right atrial pressure. By virtue of their need for inotropic support they are critically ill. Dopamine is inactivated by sodium bicarbonate solution, therefore care is required if cardiac arrest occurs, to ensure that the two drugs are not mixed.

Dobutamine

Dobutamine is a synthetic preparation very similar to dopamine but with no direct effect on the renal arteries. Any improvement in renal function seen during dobutamine administration is caused by an increase in cardiac output. Dobutamine is less likely to cause tachycardia and tachydysrhythmias. It can be safely given via a peripheral infusion if central venous access is not available. Dopamine and dobutamine are often administered concurrently to achieve a cumulative benefit on cardiac output, without the need to use potentially dangerous doses of either drug.

Patients may become highly dependent on inotropic support so interruption of the infusion must be avoided, e.g. when changing infusion solutions, or measuring the central venous pressure. Care must also be taken not to flush large quantities of the drugs into the circulation when recording the central venous pressure via a single-lumen central catheter.

Adrenaline infusions are used if other inotropic therapy has failed. Monitoring of blood glucose levels is required in addition to observations already discussed.

Isoprenaline is used occasionally as an inotropic agent when an increase in heart rate is required, i.e. in the treatment of bradydysrhythmias caused by atrioventricular block that are compromising the cardiac output and have not responded to atropine. An isoprenaline infusion may be used as an alternative to temporary pacing if the dysrhythmia proves transient, or to maintain cardiac output while a pacing wire is inserted.

NITRATES

Nitrates may be administered via several routes, sublingually, orally, transdermally or intravenously. The route and preparation selected will depend upon the speed of onset and the duration of action required.

Effects
Nitrates cause relaxation of smooth muscle leading to arterial and venous vasodilatation. This results in a reduction in the cardiac workload, by reduction in preload and afterload, and also increased myocardial perfusion by increasing coronary perfusion. Thus myocardial ischaemia, and any pain associated with it, can be relieved.

Indications
Nitrates are used primarily in the treatment of angina. They can also be effective in the treatment of cardiac failure.

Notes
Nitrates cause reduction in blood pressure, therefore careful monitoring is required – particularly when nitrates are introduced initially, and also when given intravenously. Fainting can occur, mainly when rapid-onset preparations (e.g. sublingual glyceryl trinitrate – GTN) are being used –particularly in a hot environment. Patients should be warned of this danger.

A throbbing headache is a very common side-effect of nitrate administration, probably because of cerebral artery dilatation. This may be relieved with simple analgesia but, if intolerable, the tablet being used sublingually may be spat out or swallowed, after which the drug is inactivated.

Tolerance to the nitrates will develop gradually, rendering them less effective. The exception to this is sublingual GTN the use of which can be unlimited. Education on this point is crucial since patients often think they can only use a certain amount of GTN in a day. To reduce increasing tolerance when using other nitrate preparations, a nitrate-free period is recommended every day. A break in treatment at night, by stopping oral intake in the evening and removing nitrate patches, is often most convenient unless nocturnal angina is a problem.

Administration routes

Sublingual
Nitrates given sublingually include GTN tablets and GTN spray. (Spray preparations are flammable.) These preparations have a very rapid onset (less than 1 minute) and a short effect. They are used to relieve angina, and for prophylaxis prior to undertaking any activity that the patient knows by experience will cause

angina, e.g. climbing a hill. An unlimited amount of GTN can be used; however, patients should be advised to seek medical help if a prolonged attack of angina does not respond to GTN as myocardial infarction is a possibility in any patient suffering from angina. GTN tablets have a limited shelf-life once the bottle has been opened, and fresh supplies should be obtained every 8 weeks before existing supplies are exhausted.

Oral

Oral nitrate preparations include isosorbide mononitrate and isosorbide dinitrate. Their onset of action is slower, approximately 20 minutes, and effects last up to 6 hours. Sustained-release preparations are also available to prolong the effect. If rapid relief of pain is required, isosorbide dinitrate can be chewed.

Transcutaneous

Self-adhesive patches containing GTN and GTN ointment, which is applied and then covered with an occlusive dressing, are available. If ointment is used, careful measurement of the amount applied is required. Any transcutaneous preparation must not be applied to hairy skin, when absorption may be impeded, or onto erythematous skin, when absorption may be enhanced.

In the event of cardiac arrest, nitrate patches must be removed prior to defibrillation, as there exists a risk of severe skin burning if the patch comes into contact with the defibrillator paddle.

Intravenous

Both isosorbide dinitrate and glyceryl dinitrate may be given intravenously. The solutions may be administered undiluted via a syringe driver or diluted prior to infusion. Nitrates in solution are incompatible with PVC infusion bags and giving sets, where the potency of the solution will be lost. Polyethylene syringes, infusion containers and giving sets must be used instead.

Nitrates administered intravenously may cause a profound drop of blood pressure, so very close monitoring is required.

MAGNESIUM

The role of magnesium in the treatment of patients following myocardial infarction is currently under review, in the Fourth International Study of Infarct Survival (ISIS 4) (ISIS Collaborative Group 1991). It is administered by intravenous infusion and is thought to have a protective effect on the myocardium.

FURTHER READING

Chamberlain, D., Bossaert, L., Carli, P. (1992). Guidelines for advanced life support. *Resuscitation*, **24**: 111–121.

Graver, J. (1992). Inotropes: an overview. *Intensive and Critical Care Nursing*, **8**:169–179.

Hapnes S., Robertson C. (1992). Drug delivery routes and systems. *Resuscitation*, **24**:137–142.

Henney, C.R., Dow, R.J., MacConnachie, A.M (1993). *A Handbook of Drugs in Nursing Practice*, Churchill Livingstone, London.

ISIS Collaborative Group (1991). Fourth International Study of infarct survival: Protocol for a large simple study of the effects of oral mononitrate, oral captopril an intravenous magnesium. *American Journal of Cardiology*, **68**(14): 87D–100D.

Kiess-Daily ,E. (1991). Clinical management of patients receiving thrombolytic therapy. *Heart and Lung*, **2**(5): 552–565.

Reid, J.L., Rubin, P.C., Whiting, B. (1992). *Lecture Notes on Clinical Pharmacology* (4th edn.), Blackwell Scientific Publications, Oxford.

Trounce, J. (1990). *Clinical Pharmacology for Nurses* (13th edn.), Churchill Livingstone, London.

4.

INVESTIGATING CARDIAC PATIENTS

A variety of investigations are currently available to assist in the diagnosis and management of cardiac disease. Some are performed on almost every patient with established or suspected cardiac disease. Other investigations, generally the more invasive procedures, are reserved for patients with particular problems, or those experiencing the complications of myocardial infarction.

The diagnosis of acute myocardial infarction is usually based upon three criteria:

- Clinical history.
- ECG changes.
- Elevation in blood enzyme levels.

The importance of informed consent prior to any investigative procedure cannot be overstated. Consent may be formal and documented, or informal and verbal. However, the patient must be given full and clear explanations of every investigation undertaken, unless his or her condition precludes understanding and the procedures are deemed life-saving. Explanations should then be given to the patient's relatives or friends as soon as possible.

An important consideration when patients are undergoing cardiac investigations is the potential need for psychological support and counselling after the results have been relayed to the patient. Tests that may be regarded as 'routine' by nursing and medical staff (e.g. an ECG recording), may cause considerable distress to a patient if a diagnosis of myocardial infarction is confirmed. Widespread media coverage related to many aspects of cardiac disease often results in patients having preconceptions, which may be inaccurate regarding prognosis and the impact on their lifestyle of a diagnosis of myocardial infarction.

Careful communication is required between nursing and medical staff, as well as relevant hospital departments, to ensure that the correct patient is presented for investigation at the correct time and appropriately prepared. This is particularly important for patients following myocardial infarction, where the possibility exists of sudden deterioration in the patient's condition. For this reason, investigations normally performed away from the ward environment, e.g. chest radiography and echocardiography may be performed on the ward.

This allows constant supervision of the very ill patient; it also reduces the amount of exertion required by the patient and the anxiety associated with being removed (albeit briefly) from a relatively secure and familiar environment.

If patients are taken to other departments for investigations following myocardial infarction, cardiopulmonary resuscitation equipment must be readily available and functioning. Non-nursing/medical staff must be competent in basic resuscitation procedures and aware of how to summon medical help in an emergency. Nursing staff should accompany such patients while investigations are performed. They must also be fully competent and confident in resuscitation procedures and aware of the location of emergency equipment within the department being visited.

In this chapter, some of the more usual investigations will be described:

- ECG.
- Haematological tests.
- Chest radiography.
- 24-hour ECG recording.
- Echocardiography.
- Exercise (or stress) testing.
- Right atrial pressure monitoring (for central venous pressure).
- Pulmonary artery catheterisation (Swan–Ganz catheterisation).
- Coronary angiography (cardiac catheterisation).

12-LEAD ECG

An ECG is performed upon any patient with suspected cardiac disease. It is noninvasive and requires only that the patient is able to lie still for the duration of the test. This may be a problem if the patient is in severe pain, or confused. Muscle tremor will also impair the recording. Occasionally it is necessary to shave particularly hirsute male patients in order to achieve good skin contacts with the electrodes and the patient's permission should be obtained.

If myocardial infarction is suspected or diagnosed, three serial ECGs are often recorded 1, 2 and 3 days following the onset of symptoms. This will help monitor the progression of the patient in the acute stages. The ECG may reveal:

- The cardiac rhythm and heart rate.
- The location of any ischaemic or infarcted myocardial tissue (this is achieved as conduction of electrical impulses is altered in damaged myocardium).
- Any electrode imbalance, particularly hypo- and hyperkalaemia.
- Abnormal enlargement (hypertrophy) of any of the chambers of the heart.
- The effects of some drugs, e.g. digoxin.

It must be recognised that a 12-lead ECG is required for detailed diagnosis, as recorded above. Cardiac monitoring in the acute phase of cardiac disease is initiated to allow rapid detection of changes in cardiac rhythm and cannot be relied upon for detailed diagnosis.

HAEMATOLOGICAL TESTS

Venous blood samples are analysed routinely, while a variety of tests are significant in cardiac disease.

Cardiac enzymes

Cardiac enzymes are measured, usually for 3 days in succession on days 1, 2 and 3 following the onset of symptoms, so that a pattern of results may be obtained. Infarcted myocardial tissue releases enzymes into the bloodstream and several of these can now be measured. Unfortunately, other damaged body tissues will also release enzymes, so the results are not specific to myocardial infarction. Enzyme levels are not elevated by myocardial ischaemia.

Creatine phosphokinase (CPK) is the most reliable indicator of myocardial damage. Three forms of CPK (isoenzymes) have been identified, which are released from different damaged tissues. Isoenzyme MB (CPK-MB) is the most cardiospecific. Isoenzyme MM (CPK-MM) is released from skeletal muscle and levels may be affected by intramuscular injection. Isoenzyme BB (CPK-BB) is released from nervous tissues. Separate isoenzyme levels may not be measured, since an overall measurement of CPK levels can be sufficient. Analysis of CPK-MB levels may be undertaken if the diagnosis of myocardial infarction is uncertain.

Elevation of CPK levels will occur within 72 hours of infarction, with the peak level at 24 hours. Aspartate aminotransferase (AST) is less specific and levels will rise and fall within 4–6 days, with peak levels at 24 hours. Levels of AST can also be elevated in liver disease, in shock and following intramuscular injections and defibrillation.

Lactic dehydrogenase (LDH) is also not specific to myocardial damage, levels being raised by the same causes as AST elevation, also in renal disease and haemolysis. The levels will rise and fall within 4–14 days, with a peak at 4–5 days.

Serum electrolytes

These are also measured and must be corrected if abnormal. In particular, it is important to note the potassium level as both hypo- and hyperkalaemia may cause life-threatening dysrhythmias.

Haemoglobin

The haemoglobin concentration is assessed and must be corrected if very low. This is because anaemia leads to an increase in cardiac workload. A very high haemoglobin level (polycythaemia) may be relevant since this increases blood coagulability, thus predisposing the patient to myocardial ischaemia/infarction.

Blood glucose

Blood glucose concentration is also measured. Diabetes mellitus is a predisposing factor in the aetiology of ischaemic heart disease and blood glucose levels must be stabilised. Hypoglycaemia results in an increase in adrenaline secretion, which in turn results in an increase in cardiac workload.

The erythrocyte sedimentation rate

This is raised following myocardial infarction but is not diagnostic since raised levels are seen in many inflammatory conditions.

Blood lipids

Blood lipids may also be measured; cholesterol and triglyceride levels are usually assessed. This measurement is particularly relevant in patients thought to be suffering from familial hyperlipidaemia, i.e. relatives of sufferers of that disease or patients suffering myocardial infarction at a young age. If detected, hyperlipidaemia can be treated by dietary or drug means. Therefore all family members of a confirmed case can be treated before infarction occurs, if they are at risk themselves.

To obtain accurate results of blood glucose and triglyceride levels, the patient should be starved for a given period before the blood sample is taken.

Arterial blood specimens

These may be used to assess the patient's respiratory function if hypoxia is suspected, since hypoxia may precipitate dysrhythmias and exert a negative inotropic effect on the myocardium, thus reducing cardiac output. Following cardiac arrest, arterial blood must be taken to assess the degree of metabolic acidosis (if any) that has developed as a result.

Arterial blood samples are usually obtained from the radial or femoral artery. Such arterial punctures can be quite painful and a local anaesthetic agent should preferably be used. Once the sample has been obtained, local pressure must be applied over the puncture site, to prevent haemorrhage. This is particularly important in patients with prolonged blood-clotting times, e.g. in those who have received streptokinase.

CHEST X-RAYS

Chest X-rays are performed on patients admitted with a diagnosis of chest pain, or with confirmed or suspected cardiac disease. Although a chest X-ray cannot reveal the presence or absence of myocardial ischaemia or infarction, it can yield significant information particularly with regard to:

- The size and shape of the heart, which may be significant since cardiac enlargement suggests a chronically increased cardiac workload, with the heart enlarging to compensate for this.
- Left ventricular failure, in the early stages, perhaps when the patient remains asymptomatic, distension of the pulmonary veins can be identified to allow early treatment. In more advanced left ventricular failure, pulmonary oedema can be identified in the lung fields.

A chest X-ray will also reveal the presence of dextrocardia, a rare congenital condition in which the heart lies to the right side of the chest, instead of the left. It is important that the condition is recognised immediately as the management of the patient must be changed: 12-lead ECG traces must be recorded with the position of the six chest leads reversed on the chest. If pericardial aspiration becomes necessary, knowledge of the actual position of the heart within the thorax is vital. Chest X-rays are also taken to verify the position of invasive monitoring equipment, e.g. central venous pressure lines (right atrial lines) and Swan–Ganz catheters.

Since a chest X-ray is often required early in the medical assessment of patients with heart disease, portable radiography equipment is often used. The quality of these films is not so good as films taken in the X-ray department – a factor that should be taken into account when the films are interpreted.

24-HOUR ECG RECORDING

A 24-hour ECG recording may be performed during admission, or delayed until following discharge and performed on an outpatient basis if the patient is able to understand and follow the instructions, or has available assistance.

The test is used to detect or diagnose intermittent dysrhythmias or episodes of myocardial ischaemia that have not occurred while the patient is being monitored. Some dysrhythmias are precipitated only by exercise, and these will be difficult to diagnose if the patient is resting in hospital. Three chest electrodes are attached to the patient in the normal way; these are connected to a recording device, resembling a miniature tape recorder, which is easily carried by the patient in a holster. The ECG is recorded onto electromagnetic tape, which can be analysed by computer once the test is complete.

Once the monitor is in place, the patient is asked to live normally (or as normally as possible if in hospital!) but to keep the electrodes and recorder dry. The amount of exercise undertaken may be restricted, depending on the patient's condition. While the test is in progress, the patient is asked to record all significant events in a diary. The time of waking and getting up, mealtimes, periods of exercise and type of exercise, resting, going to bed, should all be noted, with time and duration of activities. Also any symptoms experienced during the test must be documented, e.g. faintness, dizziness, chest pain, palpitations, nausea.

If the patient is unable to keep such a diary, the nursing staff must do so on their behalf. Such detailed information allows the analysis of the tape to include possible precipitating or contributory factors and to assess the impact of any ischaemia or dysrhythmias on the patient's cardiac output. Thus, appropriate treatment can be implemented, and also timed to be as effective as possible.

After 24 hours of recording the electrodes are removed, while the tape, with the patient's diary, is sent for analysis.

ECHOCARDIOGRAPHY

An echocardiogram is an ultrasound scan of the heart. As such it is a noninvasive procedure, with no documented adverse side-effects. No particular preparation or aftercare is required.

The ultrasound is performed by means of a hand-held probe, lubricated with conductive jelly (preferably warmed!) and applied to the chest. It may be necessary to reposition chest electrodes during the procedure.

Portable echocardiography equipment is available, enabling the test to be performed at the bedside of a very ill or unstable patient without the need to disturb him or her. An echocardiogram will not reveal myocardial ischaemia or infarction but is able to reveal some of the significant complications of infarction.

The overall functioning of the left ventricle can be assessed, and any areas of myocardium that have been damaged and are unable to pump adequately can be visualised (termed dyskinetic or akinetic segments).

Left ventricular aneurysms can be identified using this technique. Defects of the atrial or ventricular septum can be diagnosed, e.g. septal rupture (acquired septal defects); dysfunctioning heart valves can also be identified.

In addition, the presence of a pericardial effusion, or cardiac tamponade can be seen. Cardiac tamponade occurs when fluid, either pericardial fluid or blood, accumulates in the closed pericardial sac to such an extent that the pressure in the sac prevents normal pumping movements by the left ventricle. This causes severe compromise to cardiac output and is a cause of electromechanical dissociation at cardiac arrest. If the pressure is not relieved rapidly, death is inevitable.

EXERCISE OR STRESS TESTS

Given the psychological connotations, it is probably preferable, when discussing with patients, to refer to this investigation as an exercise test!

An exercise test records the heart's response to an increase in cardiac workload. The increase in workload is achieved by exercising the patient, usually by walking uphill on a treadmill, or cycling on an exercise bicycle. The amount of work is increased gradually on a treadmill by increasing the walking speed and uphill gradient. A variety of different protocols have been developed – known as 'staging' the exercise test. Commonly, seven stages of effort are used.

Before the test is started, a target heart rate is calculated, based on the patient's age. Electrodes are then attached to the patient and a sphygmomanometer cuff positioned, in order that the ECG, heart rate and blood pressure can be monitored continually. The test then begins with gentle exercise and the amount of effort required is increased gradually until either the test is completed, i.e. the prespecified target heart rate is reached, or symptoms develop that suggest it would be unsafe to exert the heart further, for example:

- Dyspnoea.
- Faintness.
- Hypotension.
- Dysrhythmias.

- Chest pain.
- Dizziness.
- Extreme hypertension.
- ECG evidence of ischaemia.

The exercise test is deemed positive if ECG changes reflect ischaemia, especially if this is associated with chest pain. An abnormal response in the systolic blood pressure, i.e. a drop in the systolic pressure when a slight rise might be expected in response to exercise, also constitutes a positive test result.

The stage at which the test becomes positive is significant in prognostic terms. However, false positive results are obtained, for example, from coronary artery spasm, or the effects of some drugs, e.g. digoxin.

Patient safety is an important consideration, and exercise testing is only carried out with a doctor present, in case of sudden collapse, or the development of symptoms requiring immediate treatment, e.g. dysrhythmias. Cardiopulmonary resuscitation equipment, including a range of drugs and a defibrillator must be available and functioning.

Exercise tests may be carried out shortly after an uncomplicated myocardial infarction, sometimes within 2 weeks. Exercise tests are often performed on an outpatient basis, 6–8 weeks after infarction but before the patient returns to work, if they plan to do so. An exercise test may be used to:

- Confirm a diagnosis of coronary heart disease.
- Evaluate cardiac function, and exercise capacity.
- Detect exercise related dysrhythmias.
- Indicated the prognosis following myocardial infarction.
- Evaluate treatment, by performing a series of tests.

There may also be some psychological benefit to the patient, in terms of motivation and confidence, since being able to exercise (quite strenuously if the later stages of the test can be reached) in a secure environment under medical supervision may increase the patient's confidence that normal preinfarct activities can be resumed safely, thus facilitating rehabilitation.

Most patients have few problems with exercise testing and no specific nursing care is required. Any necessary aftercare is related to the relief of any symptoms suffered by the patient and is associated with careful observation until the patient's condition stabilises.

RIGHT ATRIAL (CENTRAL VENOUS) PRESSURE MONITORING

Right atrial pressure and central venous pressure are directly related. If the venous catheter inserted for monitoring purposes is inserted into the right atrium, the right atrial pressure is recorded. If the catheter lies in the central veins outside the heart, the central venous pressure is recorded. Since there are no valves between the central veins and the right atrium, the central venous pressure will reflect the right atrial pressure (Fig. 4-1).

The right atrial pressure can be measured to provide an indication of the patient's fluid balance and also myocardial functioning. This is beneficial in the medical management of patients with low cardiac output, which may occur following myocardial infarction. Also, a right atrial catheter may be used for the administration of drugs; indeed, some drugs can only be administered safely via this route.

Once the patient's consent has been obtained, a single- or multilumen catheter is inserted into the right atrium via the antecubital, subclavian or jugular veins. Local anaesthesia and an aseptic technique are used. Owing to the negative

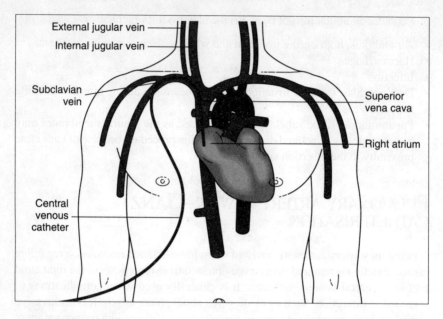

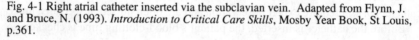

Fig. 4-1 Right atrial catheter inserted via the subclavian vein. Adapted from Flynn, J. and Bruce, N. (1993). *Introduction to Critical Care Skills*, Mosby Year Book, St Louis, p.361.

pressure (relative to atmospheric pressure) that exists in the large veins in the thorax, there is a risk of air becoming entrained into the circulation (creating a potentially fatal air embolus) during the insertion procedure. To reduce this risk, the patient is positioned lying flat with the bed tilted head down while the catheter is inserted.

Once the catheter has been positioned, it is sutured in place and a sterile dressing applied. The position of the catheter is verified by chest radiography, prior to its use. A constant flow of fluid through the catheter is required to prevent occlusion. Once the tip of the catheter is known to be positioned correctly, the right atrial pressure can be recorded with a fluid manometer, using a three-way tap. Readings are normally recorded in centimetres of water (cmH_2O). Measurements can be recorded using the mid-axillary line or the sternal notch as reference points. It is important to ensure consistency in the measurements as there is a difference in recordings obtained from the two points.

A low right atrial pressure may indicate hypovolaemia, which may cause low cardiac output unrelated to myocardial function. An increased right atrial pressure may indicate poor right ventricular function (right ventricular failure) but cannot be assumed to reflect an accurate indication of left ventricular function (as the catheter is not in the left side of the heart). Very high right atrial pressure occurs during cardiac tamponade.

Potential complications of right atrial catheterisation include:

- Air embolus, both during insertion and when replacing infusion lines etc.
- Haemorrhage.
- Infection.
- Dysrhythmias, from the irritation of the endocardium during insertion or while the catheter is *in situ*.
- Pneumothorax if the subclavian route is used as the pleural membranes may be inadvertently punctured during the insertion procedure because of their close proximity to the insertion site.

PULMONARY ARTERY (SWAN–GANZ) CATHETERISATION

A pulmonary artery catheter is inserted when more detailed information regarding cardiac function is required than can be obtained from recordings of the right atrial pressure (central venous pressure). It is generally used when complications of myocardial infarction, such as cardiogenic shock, have arisen. It is an invasive procedure, with potentially dangerous complications. Patients with pulmonary artery catheters *in situ* require expert observation and are often nursed in specialist units.

Before the catheter is inserted, the patient's blood-clotting time is checked, to ensure that an unusual risk of haemorrhage does not exist. If streptokinase has been administered to the patient, the risk of haemorrhage must be weighed against the possible benefits to the patient of potentially improved medical management. The decision is based upon the detailed information that may be obtained using the Swan–Ganz catheter. The patient's serum potassium concentration must be known and within normal limits prior to insertion, since dysrhythmias may occur during insertion and hypo- or hyperkalaemia will exacerbate the risk. Full cardiopulmonary resuscitation equipment must be available and functioning.

A multilumen catheter with an inflatable balloon just behind the distal tip is introduced into the right atrium via a large vein, usually the subclavian or internal jugular vein. The technique is similar to the insertion of a central line and precautions to prevent the introduction of an air embolus are required. Local anaesthesia and an aseptic technique should be used. Once in the right atrium, the right atrial pressure may be recorded. The balloon is then inflated (with air or carbon dioxide) and the catheter advanced through the tricuspid and pulmonary valves into a pulmonary artery. The inflated balloon facilitates this progress as it allows the catheter to 'float' in the current of circulating blood. The catheter is advanced into the smallest branches of the pulmonary artery (Fig. 4-2).

Pressure transducers attached to the catheter allow the display of pressure waveforms on monitoring equipment. These waveforms will alter as the catheter passes through the heart, reflecting the different pressure in the various chambers and blood vessels. Once in position, the catheter is secured in place and a dressing applied. A continuous flow of fluid via the catheter is maintained in order to prevent blockage. The location of the catheter is checked using chest radiography, although the position is usually clear from the pressure waveforms relayed.

The pulmonary artery catheter can then be used to record the pulmonary capillary wedge pressure. By briefly inflating the balloon in a small pulmonary

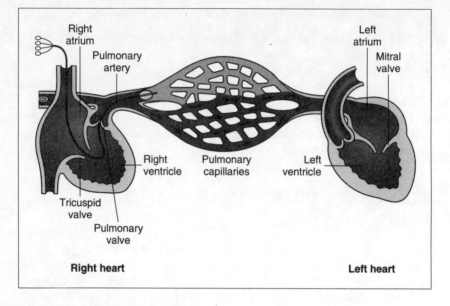

Fig. 4-2 Diagram showing the pulmonary artery in the wedge position. Adapted from Flynn, J. and Bruce, N. (1993). *Introduction to Critical Care Skills*, Mosby Year Book, St Louis, p.180.

arteriole, it is possible to block temporarily the vessel completely (termed 'wedging'), thus excluding the pressure behind the balloon in the right side of the heart. It is then possible to record the pressure at the very end of the catheter beyond the balloon; this is the pressure in the pulmonary capillary bed and is therefore referred to as the 'pulmonary capillary wedge pressure'.

This pressure is of great significance because it reflects very closely the left atrial pressure; indeed, in the normal heart the two are equal since there are no valves separating the left atrium from the pulmonary capillary bed. Thus it is possible to measure pressures on the left side of the heart, giving a far more accurate assessment of left ventricular function, which is critical in the maintenance of cardiac output. A pulmonary artery catheter can also be used to measure cardiac output directly.

Complications following the procedure include those related to central venous catheterization, namely haemorrhage, infection, air embolus, dysrhythmias and pneumothorax. Also complications may arise from 'wedging' the balloon in the pulmonary vessel. The pressure exerted during 'wedging' may rupture the pulmonary vessels, or the interruption in tissue perfusion during the procedure may lead to pulmonary infarction.

CORONARY ANGIOGRAPHY (CARDIAC CATHETERISATION)

Coronary angiography is performed to identify partially or completely occluded coronary vessels, often as a prelude to coronary artery bypass grafting. This may be performed before or after myocardial infarction. During the procedure other investigations can also be performed, e.g. the measurement of cardiac output. Remedial procedures are also possible, such as percutaneous transluminal coronary angioplasty.

Preparation for the procedure includes the signing of a formal consent and starving the patient for a minimum of 4 hours. It may be necessary to shave the skin of the groin or antecubital fossa, depending on the route to be used and the investigator's preferences. The procedure is usually carried out under local anaesthesia, although occasionally general anaesthesia is used (perhaps in the case of small children). Local anaesthesia is beneficial as the patient is able to cooperate during the procedure, by reporting symptoms such as angina. Premedication is often prescribed to reduce patient anxiety, as heightened anxiety may precipitate angina. Heart rate and rhythm are monitored throughout.

The catheter is inserted via the brachial or femoral artery and advanced into the heart. Radio-opaque dye can be injected into the coronary arteries, and radiographs taken to reveal damaged vessels. While *in situ* in partially occluded vessels, a balloon in the catheter can be inflated to reduce the occlusion, by pressure, to improve the circulation through the lumen of the vessel. This technique is known as percutaneous transluminal coronary angioplasty. The information acquired during coronary angiography enables the planning of reconstructive surgery (if this technique is possible) by means of coronary artery bypass grafting, since the exact location and extent of any occlusion(s) in the coronary arteries will be known.

Following the procedure, a variety of complications may arise:

- Haemorrhage from the arterial puncture site is possible, and regular observations of blood pressure, pulse and puncture site are required, initially every 15 minutes. The patient's mobility is restricted immediately following the procedure, especially if the femoral artery has been punctured, in order to reduce the risk of haemorrhage. The patient may be asked to remain flat in bed and to avoid bending the affected leg for several hours. A pressure dressing or sandbag may be used to prevent bleeding.
- It may be necessary to monitor the presence of peripheral arterial pulses in the artery used for the puncture, to ensure that occlusion does not occur. For example, following cardiac catheterisation via the right femoral artery, it would be appropriate to monitor the presence of the right popliteal and dorsalis pedis pulses.
- Infection may develop, and monitoring of the injection site and the body temperature will reveal this. However, some patients develop a pyrexia in response to the dye used in the procedure, although this does not usually persist.
- The patient may react to the dye injected during the procedure. The feeling of a 'hot flush' when the dye is injected is quite common and is harmless, although the patient must be warned of this possibility. Other reactions, such as headache, nausea, vomiting and skin rashes may develop during or after the procedure. Anaphylaxis may occur, usually as an immediate reaction during, rather than following, the procedure.
- Cardiac complications include angina or dysrhythmias, which must be treated in the usual way. In some cases, severe coronary artery spasm is precipitated, necessitating immediate coronary artery bypass surgery. Rarely, cardiac tamponade may occur following catheterisation, in which case, pericardial aspiration may be required.

FURTHER READING

Hampton, J.R. (1992). *The ECG Made Easy* (2nd edn.), Churchill Livingstone, London.

Hampton, J.R. (1992) *The ECG in Practice* (4th edn.), Churchill Livingstone, London.

Hopkinson, R. (1985). Using pulmonary artery catheters. *Care of the Critically Ill*, **1**(7):15–20.

Keller, S.M. (1991). Cardiovascular diagnostic techniques, in Dolan, T. (ed), *Critical Care Nursing: Clinical Management Through the Nursing Process*, F.A. Davis Company, Philadelphia., pp. 769–788.

Kiess-Daily, E. (1991). Haemodynamic monitoring, in Dolan, T. (ed), *Critical Care Nursing Nursing: Clinical Management Through the Nursing Process*. F.A. Davis Company, Philadelphia, pp. 828–854.

Miller, J. (1988). Recording central venous pressure. *Professional Nurse*, **3**(6): 188–198.

Speer, E. (1990). Central venous catheters: Issues associated with the use of single and multi-lumen catheters. *Journal of Intravenous Nursing,* **13**(1): 30–39.

Swanton, R.H. (1989). Cardiac investigations, in *Cardiology* (2nd edn.), Blackwell Scientific Publications, Oxford, pp. 377-470.

SECTION 2:

IMMEDIATE PATIENT CARE

5.

CHEST PAIN, ISCHAEMIA AND INFARCTION

Chest pain is the most common symptom experienced by individuals with coronary artery disease. While there are many different causes of chest pain, it is fortunate that pain of cardiac origin has many features that facilitate a rapid diagnosis.

PHYSIOLOGICAL CONSIDERATIONS

The heart receives its blood supply via the coronary circulation and, at rest, receives approximately 250 ml of blood every minute. Unlike other organs, the heart needs to extract the maximum amount of oxygen from the blood, about 29 ml of oxygen per minute. Consequently this means that unlike other organs, which can increase oxygen extraction as the need arises, the heart has no capacity to do this and therefore has no reserves to fall back on. The only mechanism that exists to increase oxygen supply to the heart is that of increasing blood flow, which is achieved by the action of the sympathetic nervous system, causing dilatation of the coronary arteries. Thus the balance between matching oxygen supply to oxygen demand is a very fine one and easily upset.

As with any other muscle, pain occurs if insufficient oxygen is available to meet metabolic demands. This is thought to be a result of the local accumulation of P factor, a substance that produces pain when the local concentration is high enough. In the heart this is thought to be due to the local build up of potassium and hydrogen ions. Fortunately the mechanisms involved in the transmission of pain impulses further assist in locating the source of chest pain. Visceral pain is conducted by unmyelinated C fibres, while somatic pain is carried by larger, myelinated A fibres. This produces a qualitative difference to the pain experienced, with visceral pain often described as being dull, aching and diffuse, as in angina. In contrast, somatic pain tends to be described as being sharp and well defined, the person often being able to locate the exact source of the pain.

CAUSES OF CHEST PAIN

As already mentioned, the causes of chest pain are quite numerous. However, it is useful to compare some of the more common causes, so that these can be borne in mind when assessing the individual with chest pain.

Cardiovascular causes

Cardiovascular causes of chest pain include:

- Myocardial ischaemia/infarction (MI).
- Pericarditis.
- Aortic dissection.
- Valvular disorders.
- Tachydysrhythmias.
- Anaemia.

Typically the pain of MI is described as being dull, oppressive and is often accompanied by sweating and nausea. Frequently the pain radiates down the left arm or into the jaw. The pain in ischaemia usually lasts for between 1 and 30 minutes. Pain lasting for longer than this is suggestive of infarction or unstable angina. Characteristic ECG changes often accompany chest pain of cardiac origin. In angina ST-segment depression is seen in the leads relating to the ischaemic area, and returns to normal once the pain resolves (Fig. 5-1). While following

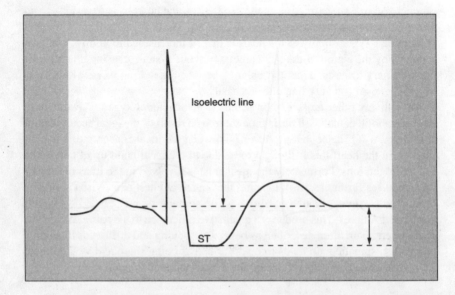

Fig. 5-1 Characteristic ECG complex with ischaemia. Adapted from Andreoli, K.G. *et al.* (1987). *Comprehensive Cardiac Care* (6th edn.), Mosby Yearbook, St Louis.

infarction ST-segment elevation is seen initially, followed by T-wave inversion and the development of pathological Q waves (Fig. 5-2). Similarly, these changes will be seen in the leads facing the infarcted area and thus help to confirm the location of the infarct. An inferior myocardial infarction is generally the result of occlusion in the right coronary artery, although a small percentage are caused by occlusion of the circumflex branch of the left coronary artery. Electrocardiographically it is demonstrated by changes in the inferior leads, namely leads II, III, and the aVF lead (Fig. 5-3).

In general, inferior infarction is considered to have a more favourable prognosis than anterior infarction; however, it is not without its characteristic complications. As the right coronary artery supplies both the SA and AV nodes in 90% of the population, it is not uncommon for the patient to develop a bradydysrhythmia or degree of heart block. Indeed, these must be looked for carefully and treatment instigated if the person becomes haemodynamically compromised. More recently it has become evident that up to one-third of patients with an inferior myocardial infarction also have some degree of right ventricular involvement. Often this passes undetected, and is generally obscured electrocardiographically by the large left ventricular muscle mass. However, it should be considered in any individual with an inferior infarct who develops haemodynamic problems, particularly hypotension associated with a raised central venous pressure. Changing the standard ECG precordial lead placement to include a set taken on the right side can assist the diagnosis, with ST-segment elevation being common in leads V3R and V4R (Fig. 5-4).

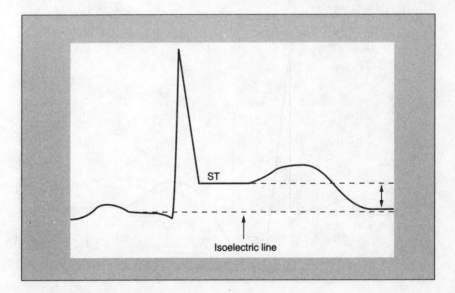

Fig. 5-2 Characteristic ECG complex following infarction. From Andreoli, K.G. *et al.* (1987) *Comprehensive Cardiac Care* (6th edn.), Mosby Yearbook, St Louis.

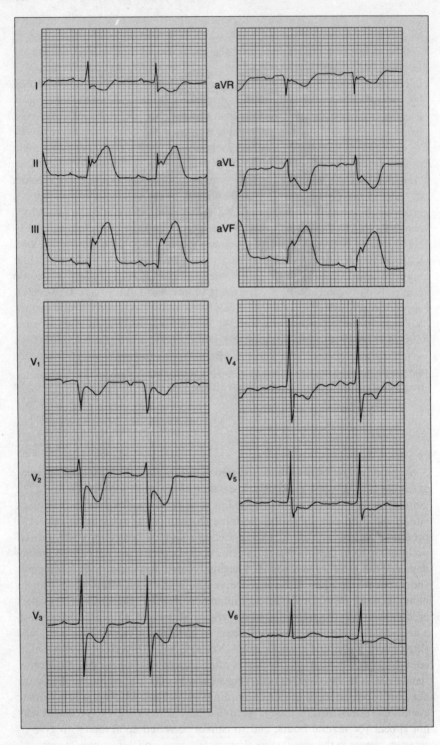

Fig. 5-3 12-lead ECG following inferior myocardial infarction.

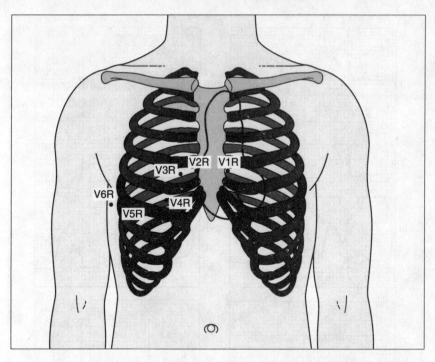

Fig. 5-4 Placement of precordial leads to detect right ventricular infarct (RVI). Character
-istic S–T elevation greater than 1mm, in V3R and V4R indicative of RVI.

Anterior infarction, and the associated anterolateral and anteroseptal infarcts, generally carry a worse prognosis. The damage is caused by occlusion of the left coronary artery, usually involving the left anterior descending branch. The exact site of the occlusion helps to determine the size of the subsequent infarct; a proximal occlusion leads to a large area of infarcted ventricle, while a distal occlusion reduces the infarct size. In general, the larger the amount of myocardium damaged the greater the associated haemodynamic problems, with cardiogenic shock occurring when 40% or more ventricle has been affected, carrying a mortality of 80–90%. Unlike inferior infarction, the ECG changes will be evident predominantly in the precordial leads, strictly V3 and V4 (Fig. 5-5). In contrast, anteroseptal infarction produces changes in leads V1–V4 (Fig. 5-6), and anterolateral infarction changes in V4–V6, aVL and I (Fig. 5-7). Thus it can be seen that, since cardiac monitoring is often carried out using a modification of standard lead II, any changes occurring anteriorly may well be missed, hence the need for repeated 12-lead ECG recordings on anyone with a possible cardiac condition. It must also be remembered that the characteristic ECG changes may not appear for several hours, and so cannot be relied upon totally to give an accurate picture in the acute stages. Fortunately myocardial infarction leads to the release of enzymes normally contained within the cardiac cells, and these may be detected in the blood to assist in the confirmation of the diagnosis.

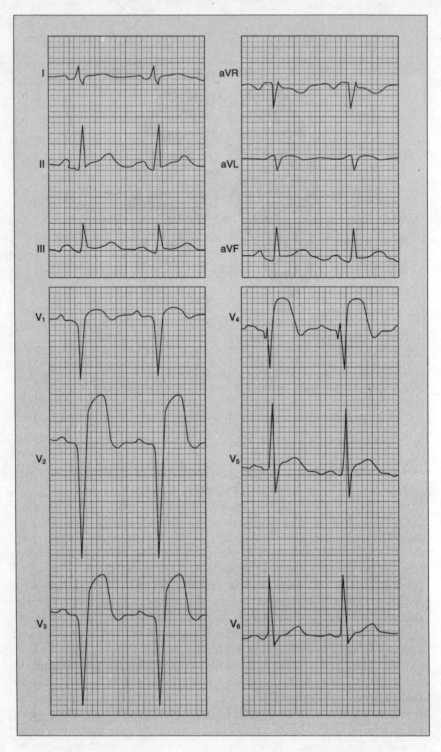

Fig. 5-5 12-lead ECG following anterior infarction.

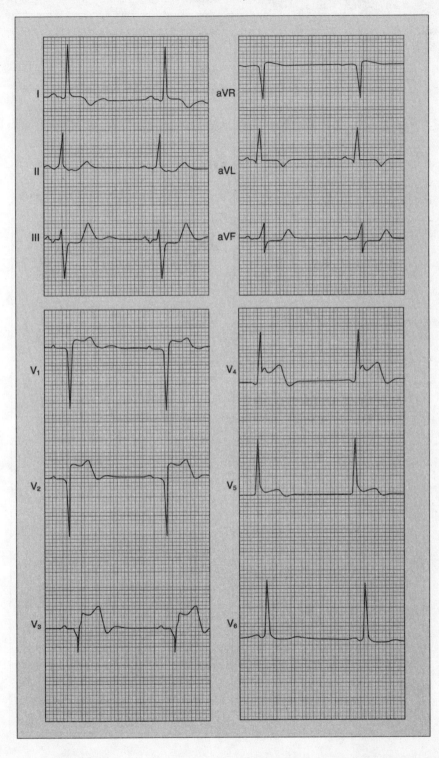

Fig. 5.6 12-lead ECG following anteroseptal infarction.

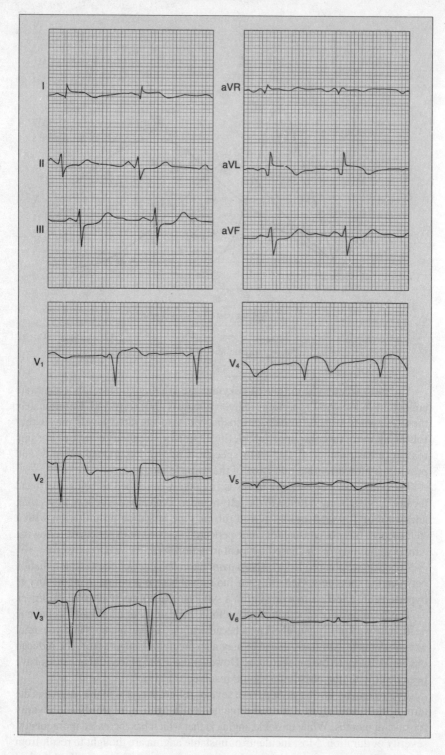

Fig. 5-7. 12-lead ECG following anterolateral infarction.

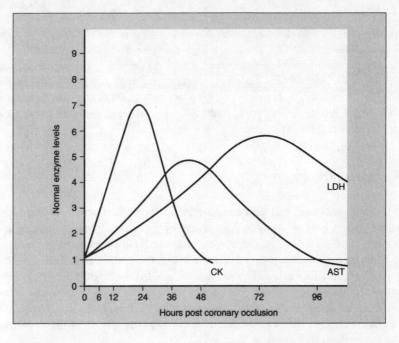

Fig. 5-8. Diagram illustrating enzyme release following infarction.

The most frequently measured enzymes are creatine kinase (CK), aspartate aminotransferase (AST) and lactic dehydrogenase (LDH) (Fig. 5-8). Unfortunately these enzymes are not totally cardiospecific, and elevated levels may occur following intramuscular injection, defibrillation or strenuous exercise. For this reason, measurement of the more specific CK-MB has gained ground, and provides a more accurate reflection of the damage incurred.

The pain produced by pericarditis is frequently described as being sharp and localised, often being referred to the left shoulder. Typically it is relieved by sitting and learning forward and a friction rub may be heard on auscultation with a stethoscope. It is not unusual for some pericardial pain to be experienced following a myocardial infarction caused by local irritation.

Aortic dissection produces a sharp pain felt in the anterior chest, with radiation between the shoulders. Generally the individual has an accompanying history of hypertension, chest trauma or Marfan's syndrome (a connective tissue disorder).

The development of a tachydysrhythmia, especially in an already ischaemic heart, may well precipitate chest pain because of the sudden increase in myocardial oxygen demand. Similarly anaemia may also precipitate angina from the reduced oxygen delivery to the myocardium. However, once the precipitating causes have been dealt with, the chest pain should resolve.

Angina can be further divided into several different types. Stable angina is the term given to anginal pain that has remained unchanged in frequency and severity for several months. While unstable angina is that which has increased in frequency, severity or duration. Most incidents of unstable angina are thought to result from rupture of an atheromatous plaque in a coronary artery. This partially detached plaque or the accompanying thrombus results in severe narrowing of the artery.

In general, newly diagnosed angina is considered as unstable until its course becomes obvious. Crescendo angina is a term sometimes used to describe a form of unstable angina where there is a high likelihood of myocardial infarction occurring at any time. The final type of angina is one that follows an atypical picture, consequently it is called atypical angina or Prinzmetal's angina. It is thought to be caused by coronary artery spasm and occurs at rest. The ECG shows ST-segment elevation, as opposed to the ST-segment depression that accompanies the more usual forms of angina.

Pulmonary causes

Pulmonary causes of chest pain comprise pleuritic irritation, pulmonary embolism and/or pneumothorax. Any disorder involving the parenchyma of the lung may produce chest pain, such as simple viral infections. However, most of the causes of chest pain from pulmonary factors involve the pleura. Classically, pain of pleural origin is exacerbated by respiration and is described typically as being one-sided, sharp and severe. Pulmonary embolism is often associated with a sudden onset of chest pain, usually accompanied by dyspnoea and tachycardia. A similar picture is seen in spontaneous pneumothorax, although the respiratory distress tends to be more acute.

Gastrointestinal causes

Gastrointestinal causes of chest pain comprise oesophageal reflux, oesophageal spasm and/or carcinoma. The pain caused by oesophageal reflux is often related to the ingestion of food, or changing to a lying down position. The pain is most likely to be described as being burning in nature and typically is substernal in location. Generally it may be relieved by antacids. However, oesophageal spasm may closely mimic the signs of angina/infarction and is often unaffected by the administration of antacids, although relieved by nitrates and calcium-channel blockers, so disguising the true nature of the pain.

Skeletal causes

Skeletal causes of chest pain comprise rib fractures, costochondritis and/or osteoarthritis. Pain produced by skeletal causes may be either sharp or dull in nature. Usually, however, it can be located specifically by the patient. A degree of skeletal pain can usually be expected following cardiopulmonary resuscitation and may prove to be quite distressing for the individual, requiring careful analgesic control.

Neurological causes

Neurological causes of chest pain comprise intercostal neuralgia and/or herpes zoster. Pain produced by these causes tends to be localised or referred according to the nerves involved. Generally there is associated tenderness along the nerve path. Herpes zoster infection becomes evident by the appearance of the characteristic reddening of the skin and a vesicular rash.

Psychogenic causes

Psychogenic causes of chest pain comprise panic attacks and/or hyperventilation. Hyperventilation causes a drop in pCO_2 from increased exhalation. This loss of acidic carbon dioxide results in alkalosis, which inhibits the dissociation of oxyhaemoglobin resulting in less oxygen being available to the tissues, including the heart.

ASSESSMENT OF THE INDIVIDUAL WITH CHEST PAIN

As already seen, the causes of chest pain are numerous and careful nursing assessment will ensure that potentially life-threatening causes are not missed and that prompt medical attention is sought. As a basic rule, any complaint of chest pain should be treated seriously and promptly reported to the medical staff so that accurate diagnosis can be made. Similarly, nursing assessment should be reduced to the absolute minimum during the acute phase and the nursing goals (in conjunction with the medical staff) directed towards establishing pain relief, identification of the nature of the pain and maintaining close patient observation. A more detailed assessment may be performed once the patient's condition has stabilised, and includes such areas as risk factors for coronary heart disease.

Several factors need to be considered in the nursing assessment, all of which can be ascertained quite quickly and in conjunction with other essential assessment, such as the monitoring of vital signs. These are outlined below.

- Description of pain. Note the patient's description of the pain, i.e. is it sharp, dull, a feeling of pressure?
- Location. Where is the pain, and does it radiate anywhere?
- Precipitating factors. What was the patient doing when the pain occurred? Was it associated with activity or rest?
- Duration. How long did the pain last for, or is it still present? What did the patient do to alleviate the pain? Did they take any medication?
- Associated symptoms. Was the pain associated with any nausea, sweating or dizziness?

As well as these specific factors, the general assessment must include the recording of vital signs, such as temperature, pulse, respiratory rate and blood pressure. These not only may reveal deviation from the normal range but serve to provide a baseline for subsequent readings. Additionally, any patient admitted with chest pain should have cardiac monitoring established, and a 12-lead ECG recorded, if local protocols allow. A calm, confident approach by the nursing team will help in reducing the inevitable anxiety experienced by the patient. Care should also be taken to ensure clear explanations of all actions are given, especially since routine observations and investigations may be quite daunting. An already anxious patient may well be bewildered by the activity around them and the seemingly endless investigations. Thus an organised team approach can do much to instill confidence.

Management

General nursing management of the individual with chest pain

All patients admitted with chest pain should be assumed to have a cardiac problem until proven otherwise. Thus they should be admitted to a bed that permits close visual observation and equipment should be available to establish continuous cardiac monitoring. Resuscitation equipment needs to be immediately available, should life-threatening dysrhythmias become evident. Ideally, the nursing staff present should be able to interpret accurately cardiac rhythms and be sufficiently experienced to provide adequate resuscitation skills, including defibrillation. A brief nursing assessment will provide vital information in helping to determine the exact nature of the chest pain and provide a valuable baseline against which subsequent assessments can be compared. Informing the medical staff of the patient's arrival should be a priority, so that prompt pain relief can be instigated, and the necessary investigations started. These will almost certainly include 12-lead ECG, chest radiography (usually portable), routine blood tests for concentrations of urea and electrolytes, plus cardiac enzymes. Other investigations to assist in the confirmation of a diagnosis will be performed as thought necessary by the medical staff, e.g. a V/Q scan may be ordered if a differential diagnosis of pulmonary embolism is being considered. Once again, the nursing staff must ensure that clear explanations of any proposed investigations are given to the patient and their verbal consent obtained. More specific nursing management is required once the exact nature of the chest pain has been confirmed.

Management of the individual with angina

Patients with established stable angina mainly require nursing interventions in relation to three areas: understanding the angina, general coping advice and specific drug knowledge. These may be offered by nurses in either the acute hospital setting or the primary health care team; however, clear communication channels need to be established to prevent the confusion that can arise from conflicting advice. In general, patients accept the cause of angina and understand the basic problem of oxygen supply and demand; however, the severity of the psychological reactions to the diagnosis should never be underestimated, and patients and their families frequently need help to move on from this crisis.

General coping advice that should be given includes general measures to improve cardiovascular fitness, such as smoking cessation, maintenance of ideal body weight and the taking of regular exercise (although patients should be advised to exercise up to the point of chest pain and never to go beyond). On a similar theme, care should be taken not to engage in strenuous activity during cold weather or following a heavy meal. In most individuals with stable angina, the mainstay of treatment consists of drug therapy to relieve or prevent the symptoms of angina. The main types of drugs used consist of nitrates, beta blockers and calcium-channel antagonists. It is essential that the individual fully understands the action and correct use of their medication so that they may obtain maximum benefit. To this end, it goes without saying that the nurse must also have a full knowledge, in order to be in a position to help the patient. More specific advice will be needed in relation to any cardiac investigations that the patient undergoes, such as exercise testing, coronary arteriography or coronary angioplasty, and to ensure that the advice or interventions being suggested are appropriate for that person's circumstances.

Management of the individual with myocardial infarction/unstable angina

Since there is a high likelihood of unstable angina proceeding to myocardial infarction, the nursing strategies employed are identical to those used following myocardial infarction. In unstable angina, intravenous infusions of a nitrate (e.g. glyceryl trinitrate) may be used to provide pain relief, with the dose titrated against the patient's response. Care is needed that the amount given does not seriously affect arterial blood pressure and cardiac output. Thus the individual receiving intravenous nitrates should ideally have continuous blood pressure monitoring.

As well as the more general measures already outlined, the specific goals of nursing care are: to ensure adequate pain relief; to reduce myocardial oxygen demand and size of infarct; to reduce anxiety and circulating catecholamines; and to detect rapidly any change in status. Throughout the acute phase, effective communication must be maintained with the patient and his or her family. This includes being honest and not offering false encouragement. There are many anecdotal accounts of nurses minimising the seriousness of the patient's condition, only to have to deal with the sudden death of that individual later on.

Pain relief is best achieved by the administration of intravenous diamorphine, with antiemetic cover. This will also assist in reducing anxiety and so reduce catecholamine circulation, as well as producing a degree of vasodilation, which will reduce preload. Oxygen therapy may be prescribed and the usual cautions must be observed, particularly if the patient has a chronic respiratory problem. The provision of analgesia should be an ongoing concern and the medical staff informed if the prescribed drugs are not providing total pain relief.

Reduction in infarct size is achieved by restoring coronary patency by the routine use of thrombolytic agents, generally streptokinase given intravenously. Close observation of the patient receiving thrombolytic therapy is required, with particular attention given to the possibility of reperfusion dysrhythmias (e.g. bradycardias or accelerated idioventricular rhythm) and sensitivity occurring. Following thrombolytic therapy, the patient is at increased risk of a bleeding disorder, which presents additional problems should the need arise for invasive procedures such as the insertion of a central venous catheter or temporary pacing wire. Reduction in myocardial oxygen demand is achieved by the use of enforced bedrest and nursing assistance with activities of living. The use of a commode as opposed to a bedpan is preferred as it requires a lower oxygen consumption. However, a balance must be achieved between provoking unnecessary anxiety by over-zealous nursing intervention and putting the patients at risk by allowing them to exert themselves too much.

The rapid detection of deterioration in the patient's condition is facilitated by the intelligent use of observation skills, assisted by techniques such as cardiac monitoring particularly noting dysrhythmias and falling cardiac output. (The risk of dysrhythmias developing falls off as time elapses.) The accurate monitoring of fluid balance, preferably by daily weighing, can alert the nurse to the development of cardiac failure. General recording of vital signs should be performed as often as the patient's condition warrants, with the general trend in the readings being more important than a 'one-off' reading. Again care should be taken that the recording of observations should not take over and time should be allowed for the patient to rest. To aid in this the use of automatic blood pressure recorders are advisable in someone who requires particularly close monitoring.

The degree of observation and nursing intervention may be decreased as the patient's condition stabilises; however, any change from the expected recovery path needs to be evaluated carefully. For example the re-emergence of chest pain in someone after a myocardial infarction should be treated seriously and the medical staff informed as it may signify reinfarction or extension of the existing infarct. Should this happen then the interventions used in the acute phase should be reinstituted until the patient's condition stabilises again. The devastating effect this can have on the patient and their families should not be overlooked. The patient has been receiving information on returning back to normal and suddenly is back to 'square one'. It should be emphasised, however, that many patients make an uneventful recovery following myocardial infarction and, with informed nursing care, those that run into problems may be offered a better chance of survival and be assisted through the rehabilitation phase.

FURTHER READING

Altice, N.F., Jamison, G. B. (1989). Interventions to facilitate pain management in myocardial infarction. *Journal of Cardiovascular Nursing*, **3**(4): 49–56.

Green, E. (1992). Solving the puzzle of chest pain. *American Journal of Nursing*, **92**(1):32–37.

Herlitz, J., Richter, A., Hjalmarson, A. , Holmberg, S. (1986). Variability of chest pain in acute myocardial infarctions. *International Journal of Cardiology*, **13**(1):9–26.

Messineo, F. C., Hager W. D. (1989). Hemodynamic complications of acute myocardial infarction. *Hospital Practice*, **24**(8):147–164.

Rossi, L. Leary E. (1992). Evaluating the patient with coronary artery disease. *Nursing Clinics of North America*, **27**(1):171–188.

Smith, C. E. (1988). Assessing chest pain quickly and accurately. *Nursing*. **18**(5), 52–60.

Thompson, C. (1989). The nursing assessment of the patient with cardiac pain on the coronary care unit. *Intensive Care Nursing*, **5**(4):147–154.

6.

CARDIOGENIC SHOCK – NURSING IMPLICATIONS

John is a 63-year-old solicitor who you nursed 2 years ago when he was admitted to the ward with an anterior myocardial infarction (MI). He has now been admitted with further chest pain and anterior lateral changes on his ECG.

You sense he seems a little restless and agitated – he says he 'doesn't feel right'. John seems to be breathing faster and as you hold his hand it seems cool and sweaty. As you talk with him and check his blood pressure, you notice that he looks paler and his face and lips look blue. His blood pressure has dropped to 80/65 mmHg and his cardiac monitor is showing a sinus tachycardia of 120 beats/minute with numerous multifocal ventricular ectopics.

You alert John's doctor and he tells you John is going into cardiogenic shock. What does this really mean? What changes will you have to consider making in the assessment, planning, intervention and evaluation processes in John's care?

DEFINITION

Cardiogenic shock results from the inability of the heart to pump effectively. When the pumping ability of the heart fails, there is a reduced blood flow to the body's tissues, which causes inadequate oxygen and nutrient delivery to the cells. This disrupts normal cellular metabolism and triggers the body response to shock. Cardiogenic shock is traditionally defined as a:

- Systolic blood pressure less than 85 mmHg or mean arterial blood pressure less than 65 mmHg.
- Cardiac index less than 2.2 litres/minute/m^2.
- Elevated pulmonary artery wedge pressure greater than 18 mmHg.

All these indices demonstrate a failing heart with an inadequate cardiac output. Important patient assessment pointers to inadequate cardiac output include :

- Rapid, thready pulse.
- Arrhythmias.
- Oliguria.
- Decreased level of consciousness.

The gravity of a patient developing cardiogenic shock cannot be overstated. Acute MI is the most common precipitating factor; up to 15% of all patients admitted to hospital with an acute MI will die from cardiogenic shock and most will have damage to at least 40% of the myocardium. Patients at greatest risk of developing this complication are those who have sustained an anterior or anterior septal MI, caused by an obstruction to the left anterior descending artery, which supplies the largest area of the myocardium. The stark fact is that the mortality from cardiogenic shock remains high at approximately 90%, most of these patients die within 24 hours of the cardiac insult, few survive more than 4 days.

Cardiogenic shock can also be precipitated by:

- Arrhythmias, e.g. severe tachyarrhythmias or bradyarrhythmias where cardiac output is ineffective.
- Cardiac tamponade – blood collecting in the pericardial sac and causing and obstruction of the ventricular function. This can occur after cardiac surgery or from trauma, e.g. knife injury.
- End-stage cardiomyopathy.
- Valvular disease, e.g. acute aortic regurgitation causing the left ventricle to fail.

STAGES OF CARDIOGENIC SHOCK

The response of the patient to shock is unique to that individual; it is dependent on the severity and duration of the shocked state together with any coexisting problems. It can generally be characterised into three stages.

Stage 1

In the early or compensatory stage the sympathetic nervous system (SNS) responds to the insult/injury in an attempt to compensate for the reduced cardiac output (CO). This is achieved by increasing heart rate (chronotropism), heart force (inotropism), stroke volume and by causing selective vasoconstriction; as a result the skin becomes cool and clammy. The reduction in renal blood flow/pressure stimulates the juxtaglomerular apparatus in the walls of the afferent arterioles to release renin. Through several chemical interactions this is converted into angiotensin II, a potent vasoconstrictor. Evidence of this can be seen in the clinically shocked, peripherally 'shut-down' patient.

The adrenal cortex responds to angiotensin II by releasing aldosterone, which, together with the antidiuretic hormone (ADH), increases the reabsorption of sodium and water by the renal tubules. Owing to the decreased renal perfusion the urine output is diminished and may become less than 20 ml/hour; urea, creatinine and nitrogen are retained, as indicated by rising blood levels and the risk of acute tubular necrosis and acute renal failure exists.

Additionally, in response to a developing hypoxic state, the aortic and carotid chemoreceptors respond to the decreased oxygen tension by increasing the rate and depth of respirations.

Stage 2

In the middle (progressive) state the compensatory mechanisms fail to maintain an adequate output. Under these conditions anaerobic metabolism takes place and metabolic acidosis develops. This causes arteriolar vasodilation and venule constriction. Stagnant hypoxia results, further exacerbating the cellular disturbances as demonstrated by cardiac dysrhythmias. Oedema occurs as a result of a fluid shift from the dilated capillaries to the interstitial spaces. Protein also leaks through the enlarged capillary pores, resulting in a lowered serum osmotic pressure and causing fluid shift and the continued development of oedema.

Cardiac contractility is impaired by the effect of the myocardial depressant factor (MDF), which is released by the ischaemic pancreas, and this contributes to the further deterioration of circulation and cardiac output. To compensate, the heart rate continues to increase but during the later stages may become weaker and irregular (dysrhythmic). The pulse pressure decreases because of a rise in diastolic pressure (from increased peripheral vascular resistance) and a decrease in systolic pressure (from decreased stroke volume). Left (pulmonary capillary wedge) and right (central venous) filling pressures rise because of ineffective clearance/pumping of the blood from the heart. This leads to the development of pulmonary oedema in the lungs and the resultant clinical patient observations of, for example, cyanosis and tachypnoea. There is further congestion of organs whose venous blood feeds back into the heart, e.g. kidneys, liver, brain and peripheral tissues.

Stage 3

In the late (refractory) stage of shock the compensatory mechanisms have failed totally and the reduced tissue perfusion and prolonged compensatory vasoconstriction leads to increased cellular and, ultimately, organ dysfunctioning. The cardiac output continues to reduce as a result of the decreased coronary blood supply and the presence of acidosis and toxins. The blood pressure falls as the cardiac output decreases from a failing Starling mechanism, i.e. the myocardial fibres have been stretched beyond their optimal length and are ineffective to eject blood. Respiratory failure, poor ventilation and carbon dioxide retention leads to respiratory acidosis, which adds to the metabolic acidosis already present. In addition, this provides a suitable respiratory environment for atelectasis and consolidation to develop.

Tissue and organ perfusion is further compromised by disseminated intravascular coagulation (DIC), which develops with the stagnation of capillary blood and the ensuing clumping of erythrocytes and platelets. With this, the blood-clotting factors are consumed by the widespread microcoagulation and the fibrin clots break down.

Cardiac and respiratory failure lead to further depression of all cerebral functions. Early signs are restlessness, apprehension and confusion; later, listlessness, apathy and unconsciousness occur as cerebral hypoxia increases. The irreversible stage of shock progresses to failure of all body systems and ultimately, to death.

These patients are extremely ill (Fig. 6-1) and dependent on the nurse for meeting all their needs. It is important therefore that throughout the total care given to the patient and their family, that proficiency in both the science and the art of nursing should be demonstrated – one area must not be negated at the expense of the other.

Since cardiogenic shock is such a serious complication, the optimum nursing care that can be achieved is one that builds in prevention and early detection

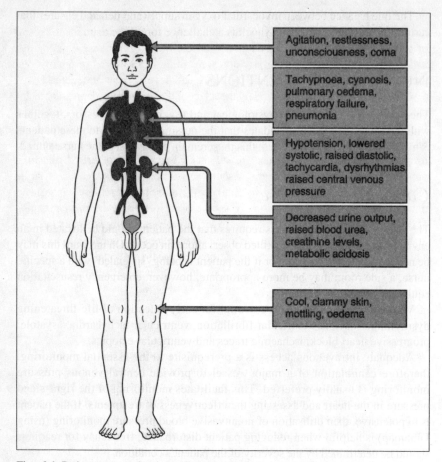

Agitation, restlessness, unconsciousness, coma

Tachypnoea, cyanosis, pulmonary oedema, respiratory failure, pneumonia

Hypotension, lowered systolic, raised diastolic, tachycardia, dysrhythmias, raised central venous pressure

Decreased urine output, raised blood urea, creatinine levels, metabolic acidosis

Cool, clammy skin, mottling, oedema

Fig. 6-1 Patient presentation in cardiogenic shock.

measures. Despite all the preventative measures available, e.g. prompt assessment and treatment of dysrhythmias, haemodynamic disturbances, minimising infarction size (through beta blockers and vasodilators) and maximising reperfusion (through thrombolysis), the outcome of cardiogenic shock is determined predominantly by early and effective treatment through assessment and intervention.

In essence, the primary aim of both nursing and medical treatment is to influence the four main factors that affect cardiac output:

1. Preload: the amount of blood left in the ventricles at the end of diastole. This should be sufficient to stretch the myocardial fibres to eject blood into the aorta but not enough to over-stretch beyond optimum (Starling's curve).
2. Afterload: the resistance against which the heart must pump. This is basically referring to the degree of arteriolar tone (systemic vascular resistance) present in the vascular system. Obviously, a degree of resistance is needed to maintain blood pressure but not too much otherwise the heart has to work hard to eject out against that force.
3. Contractility.
4. Heart rate.

The fine balance between myocardial oxygen supply and demand ensures that caring for those in cardiogenic shock is a challenge for all the team.

NURSING INTERVENTIONS

The vital interplay between physiological and psychological stressors, together with the severe prognosis, mandates that the nursing care given to these patients is truly holistic and individualised; this must remain uppermost in the nurse's mind.

Cardiovascular care

The critical nature of the illness requires that the patient should be located in an environment where close and skilled observation can occur. On the ward this may be near to the nursing station, or if the patient is being 'specialed' with a specific nurse, a side room may be more appropriate; however, emergency resuscitation equipment should be at hand.

Vital cardiac monitoring is essential for early detection of life-threatening dysrhythmias such as ventricular fibrillation, ventricular tachycardia, asystole, progressive heart block, ischaemic traces and ventricular ectopics.

Adequate intravenous access is a prerequisite to the essential monitoring, therefore cannulation of a major vessel to provide central venous pressure monitoring is usually preferred. This facilitates monitoring of the right-sided pressure in the heart and assessing the effectiveness of treatments. If the patient is hypotensive, then utilisation of noninvasive blood pressure monitoring (using Dinamap) is helpful when reducing patient disturbance; frequency for readings should be determined by the severity of the patient's condition.

It is important that when assessing, planning, implementing and evaluating care that all therapeutic measures are analysed in relation to the factors that affect cardiac output. The following are key therapies.

Volume replacement
Approximately 20% of patients may be hypovolaemic from poor fluid intake, aggressive diuretic therapy etc. Fluid challenges may be prescribed of 100/200 ml over 10–20 minutes. Following this, close monitoring of the central venous pressure and urine output is essential (urinary catheterisation is imperative).

Vasodilator therapy
Vasodilators act to combat the increased vascular resistance that is resultant from the selective vasoconstriction. The most commonly used vasodilators include GTN and isosorbide dinitrate.

Inotropic therapy
Inotropic therapy is used to increase (strengthen) myocardial contractility. Dobutamine is a popular inotrope in that it can be safely administered through a peripheral line. As with all inotropic drugs, the therapeutic regime is dose-related; it is therefore important that the nurse can calculate micrograms/kilogram/minute

in order to titrate and achieve optimum parameters. Dopamine is an inotropic agent with specific renal and cardiac dose-related ranges. Adrenaline, a more potent inotropic agent, can be used as an infusion in those most severely affected by cardiogenic shock. For this reason, it is primarily utilised within the critical care areas where more invasive monitoring is available.

Diuretic therapy
Diuretics are drugs that reduce preload and pulmonary/systemic congestion through a diuresis of water and solutes. This eases breathing and decreases myocardial work and oxygen requirement. The key diuretic in use is frusemide, a potent loop diuretic whose peak action can be seen within 30 minutes if administered intravenously. However, diuretics can cause severe electrolyte imbalance, particularly of potassium, which may precipitate cardiac dysrhythmias. Hypovolaemia and hypotension may also result. In less acute management situations, thiazide and potassium-sparing diuretics can be used. Other drugs that may be used, e.g. antiarrhythmics and digoxin, are also part of the therapeutic regimes to maximise cardiac output by optimising preload, afterload, cardiac contractility and heart rate.

Nursing responsibility in this area of care focuses on the action and side-effects of the key pharmaceutical treatments. Close monitoring of all vital signs is imperative because of dramatic changes in cardiovascular status in response to inotropic administration. It is essential that vasodilatory and inotropic therapy is continuous and weaned gradually. Meticulous observation with documentation of all cardiovascular, respiratory and urinary parameters is essential, and reporting of the patients progress is central to the multidisciplinary approach to care.

Respiratory care

Immediate attention is given to optimising the oxygen level in the blood (pO_2). Humidified oxygen is administered via a face mask or, if not tolerated, nasal cannulae. Blood gas analysis will be performed to establish the effectiveness of oxygenation and to determine whether a higher percentage of oxygen is required. The main nursing responsibilities in this area focus on ensuring that there is continuous oxygen administered, upright posturing as condition allows and encouragement of breathing exercises to discourage lung consolidation. Skilled nursing will be required to develop a trust relationship to ensure that continuous oxygen is being taken, particularly if the patient is becoming hypoxic and cardiac output is affecting cerebral blood flow. It is not only important to improve arterial oxygenation and thereby reduce myocardial workload but also to ensure that arterial blood gas analysis and subsequent treatment changes will reflect the oxygen percentage prescribed.

No matter how complex the patient care is becoming, it is also important to ensure that firm pressure is applied over an arterial stab site for approximately 10 minutes to ensure that haematoma formation does not occur. If frequent sampling is occurring, not only can this be extremely painful to the patient, it can only be indicative of a deteriorating clinical picture and full patient assessment should occur to review patient problems and the future direction to be taken. A deterioration may indicate the need for continuous positive airways pressure or intubation and ventilation. The later will necessitate a transfer to an intensive care unit.

Nutritional needs

Owing to the experienced lethargy, tachypnoea and possible hepatic engorgement from right-sided failure, nutritional needs are not a focus of care at this time. Any meals/fluids taken should be as tolerated by the patient and made as nutritious and appetising as possible. As other systems improve, the appetite will return to normal. It is only in later stages of resolving cardiogenic shock that, if this problem continues, enteral/parenteral means of feeding will be considered.

Renal care

A urinary catheter must be *in situ* in a patient in cardiogenic shock who is receiving active treatment. In the acute stage, hourly measurements must be monitored and reported. This is particularly relevant in light of treatment changes, e.g. diuretic administration. Potassium levels will need to be monitored and supplements may be ordered to correct a hypokalaemic state or measures to reduce the serum potassium if renal function is deteriorating (e.g. administration of calcium resonium).

Hygiene care

In order to meet the patient's hygiene needs and not increase myocardial oxygen demand, there needs to be appropriate planning of all aspects of care. All therapeutic and nursing actions must be organised to permit uninterrupted rest periods. This necessitates that the nurse is well-organised in planning nursing care, and can advocate on behalf of the patient in organising other aspects of treatments, e.g. X-rays, physiotherapy, blood tests, visitors.

Although rest is necessary to decrease the patient's energy demands, complications such as deep vein thrombosis, joint contractures and chest infections must be prevented. It is important that all essential nursing care is directed by the needs and tolerance of the individual patient.

The cardiac patient will particularly need effective pressure area care. The presence of dependent oedema, which is most likely to be present, will impair skin integrity and perfusion. Appropriate assessment and use of pressure-relieving devices is essential for comfort. In addition, the continuous oxygen administration is very drying to the buccal mucosa and therefore effective mouth care is needed. If the patient is in the latter stages of cardiogenic shock, they will be cool and sweaty. Plasters and chest electrodes will be prone to slipping off and need to be checked. The use of plastic dressing spray on the skin may provide a more secure hold. Quick sponging to freshen but not tire or cool these patients is usually much appreciated. It also provides 'socially acceptable' touch – an essential part of care that can be easily overlooked within the demanding nature of this patient's total care.

Mental/psychological care

Assessment of the patients mental status is crucial in care. Not only does it provide assessment of cerebral perfusion and therefore cardiac output but it gives insight into the patient's 'coming to terms' with the illness.

Anxiety aggravates respiratory distress and increases catecholamine secretion and metabolic demands. Physical pain also increases anxiety and therefore metabolic demands, so every effort should be made for accurate assessment and prompt and effective relief of pain. Through building up a relationship with the patient, the nurse can take time to identify the patient's concerns and, where possible, provide honest explanations, demonstrating at all times dignity and respect for the patient.

Some attempt must be made to establish a degree of 'normality'; from consideration for day/night continuity, enabling patient participation and control of care, to encouraging 'sensitive' family/friend visiting. With visiting, all should appreciate and respect that visits must be adjusted according to the patient's condition/wishes.

Shock, of any classification, is a critical and life-threatening condition and creates fear and anxiety in the patient. In this situation, the patient experiences loss of privacy and independence. What it means to the patient and the effect of his or her fear and concerns on his or her condition should never be underestimated.

Family/friend care

Family and friends need support at this stressful time. There may be an inability to cope with the situation and deal with the severity of the prognosis, an inability to communicate with the patient or each other, or a total feeling of helplessness. The nurse must remember that each person will deal differently with this situation.

In any communication with the family there should be realistic honest information regarding the prognosis, treatment and progression made. Specific time must be made to listen and answer truthfully their questions, either with the patient or in a private area. Any individual or family strengths can be identified and utilised to cope with this situation. Any support mechanisms that the family usually use can be organised to assist. Feelings of powerlessness may be addressed through involvement in care if the patient is consenting.

A positive nurse–patient relationship provides a basis for establishing trust and confidence. The presence of a supportive nurse and the provision of opportunities to talk will assist both the patient and the family to come to terms with the illness and potential outcomes. It is here that the expert use of interpersonal skills can make such an impact in the care: through sharing in their happy times and being with them in their sad times.

Direction of care

There may come a point in treatment where a decision is made that more invasive and aggressive treatment is required. At this point the patient is usually transferred to a critical care area where further invasive monitoring may commence (e.g. insertion of a pulmonary artery catheter) and further pharmaceutical or mechanical cardiac support measures (e.g. ventilation equipment or an intra-aortic balloon pump) may be introduced. Equally, because of the poor prognosis, the nurse must be prepared to modify the nursing care away from the use of invasive technologies towards supporting the patient (and family) towards a dignified and peaceful death.

CONCLUSION

Caring for the patient in cardiogenic shock is a stressful and challenging time for all. Owing to the critical nature of the problem, it is imperative that the nurse has sound knowledge on which to base patient care and make quality nursing decisions within the multidisciplinary approach. It is only through a collaborative approach to care that effective treatment can be given.

To maximise the potential of patient recovery, the nurse must assess skilfully, be proactive in planning and be informed in the implementation of care. Further evaluation then dictates the direction of treatment. Despite the complexity of needs and therapies required, the place of the patient within the wider family context must not be forgotten.

To perform the above and meet the needs of the patient and the family, to acknowledge respect, dignity and privacy for all, at all times, is the essence of nursing such patient. The key features for the treatment of cardiogenic shock are as follows:

- Prevention is the best form of treatment for cardiogenic shock.
- The nurse must understand the treatments and their effects on cardiac function to care skilfully for the patient.
- All 'therapies' must be considered and individualised so that cardiac function is not compromised.
- Owing to the severe prognosis, an honest, supportive and truthful relationship must be established with the patient and their family.
- Multidisciplinary teamwork is essential to effectively care for these patients.

FURTHER READING

Carolan, J. (1986). *Shock: A Nursing Guide*, Wright and Sons, Bristol.

Darovic, G.O. (1987). *Haemodynamic Monitoring Invasive and Noninvasive Clinical Application*, W B Saunders, Philadelphia.

Nurse Review (1988). *Vascular Problems*, Springhouse, Philadelphia.

Thompson, D, Webster, R (1992). *Caring for the Coronary Patient*, Butterworth-Heinemann, Oxford.

Underhill, S.L., Woods, S.L., Froelicher, E.S.S., Halpenny, C.J. (1989). *Cardiac Nursing* (2nd edn.), J B Lippincott, Philadelphia.

7.

BRADYCARDIA

Bradycardia may be defined as a heart rate below 60 beats/minute in an adult. Types of bradycardia include:

- Sinus bradycardia.
- Junctional bradycardia.
- Bradycardia associated with AV block.

Causes of bradycardia include:

- Extreme cardiovascular fitness (usually athletes).
- Hypoxia.
- Myocardial ischaemia.
- Myocardial infarction.
- Hypertension.
- Hyperkalaemia.
- Pain.
- Drug therapy (e.g. digoxin, beta blockers, lignocaine).
- Stimulation of the vagus nerve (e.g. per rectum examination, endotracheal suctioning, the Valsalva manoeuvre performed inadvertently while straining at stool or vomiting).
- Carotid sinus massage.

Other causes are not directly related to the cardiovascular system but may be relevant if they coexist with cardiac disease:

- Hypothermia.
- Hypothyroidism.
- Raised intracranial pressure.

SINUS BRADYCARDIA

Sinus bradycardia has many causes. It is often associated with a normal cardiac output and may have no clinical significance. In some circumstances, sinus bradycardia precedes life-threatening dysrhythmias and should alert the nurse to the possibility of developing complications.

Sinus bradycardia (Fig. 7-1) is characterised by normal PQRST complexes, normal P–R interval, with a regular rate below 60 beats/minute.

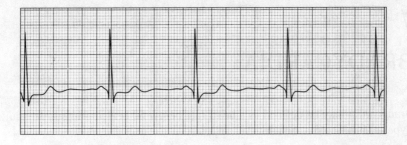

Fig. 7-1 ECG in sinus bradycardia. Adapted from Conover, M. B.(1994). *Pocket Guide to Electrocardiography* (3rd edn.), Mosby-Year Book, St Louis, p. 26.

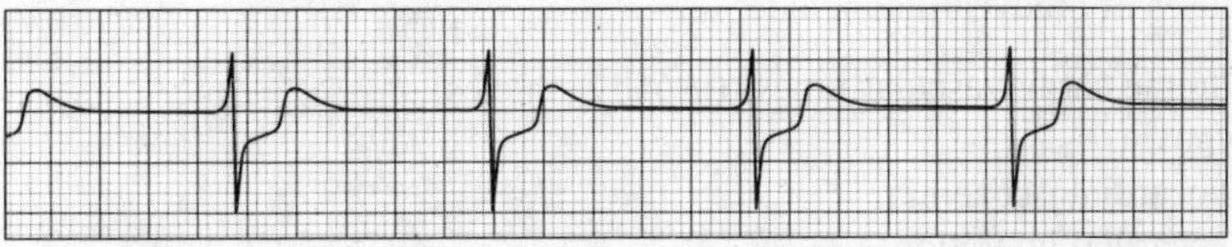

Fig. 7-2 ECG in junctional bradycardia. Adapted from Conover, M.B. (1994). *Pocket Guide to Electrocardiography* (3rd edn.), Mosby-Year Book, St Louis, p. 58.

JUNCTIONAL BRADYCARDIA

A junctional bradycardia originates from a focus in the AV node and may indicate damage to the conduction system in the heart, if following myocardial infarction. If the heart rate initiated by the SA node is greatly reduced for some reason, a junctional rhythm may supervene at a faster rate.

Junctional bradycardia (Fig. 7-2) is characterised by a normal QRST complex, with no visible P wave, or a P wave visible within the QRST complex, rather than preceding the complex. Heart rate is regular and below 60 beats/minute.

ATRIOVENTRICULAR BLOCK (HEART BLOCK)

Atrioventricular block is subdivided into three categories, depending on the severity of the disruption of the normal conductive mechanisms of the heart between the atria and the ventricles. It may result from myocardial infarction, although drug therapy (especially digoxin toxicity) or inflammatory cardiac disease (e.g. myocarditis) may be the cause.

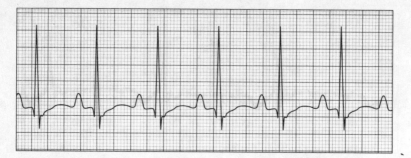

Fig. 7-3 ECG in first-degree AV block. From Conover, M.B. (1994). *Pocket Guide to Electrocardiography* (3rd edn.), Mosby-Year Book, St Louis, p. 110.

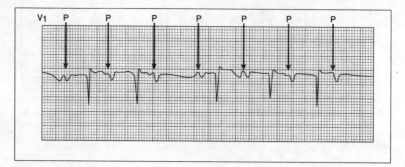

Fig. 7-4 ECG in second-degree AV block Mobitz type 1. From Conover, M.B. (1994). *Pocket Guide to Electrocardiography* (3rd edn.), Mosby-Year Book, St Louis, p. 112.

First-degree heart block

First-degree block reflects a delay in atrioventricular conduction, although each atrial impulse results in ventricular contraction. First-degree block (Fig. 7-3) is characterised by a normal PQRST complex but a prolonged P–R interval, that is, a P–R interval greater than 0.2 seconds. The heart rate is regular. First-degree block may persist, resolve or (rarely) deteriorate into second- or third-degree block.

Second-degree heart block

In second-degree block there is intermittent failure of atrioventricular conduction, i.e. some atrial impulses are not followed by ventricular contractions. There are two types of second-degree block, Mobitz type I and Mobitz type 2.

Mobitz type 1
In Mobitz type 1 second-degree block (Fig. 7-4) the P–R interval lengthens progressively until a ventricular beat is missed (or dropped) completely. This is called the Wenckebach phenomenon. The QRST complexes that occur are normal and the heart rate is irregular as the P–R interval is variable.

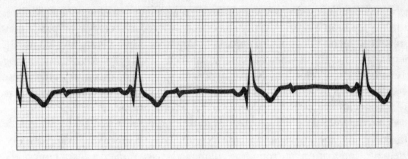

Fig. 7-5 ECG in second degree AV block Mobitz type 2. Adapted from Conover, M.B. (1994). *Pocket Guide to Electrocardiography* (3rd edn.) Mosby-Year Book, St Louis, p. 115.

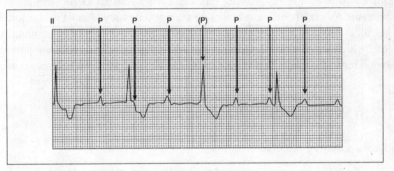

Fig. 7-6 ECG in third-degree atrioventricular block (complete heart block). Adapted from Conover, M.B. (1994). *Pocket Guide to Electrocardiography* (3rd edn.), Mosby-Year Book, St Louis, p. 116.

Mobitz type 2

In Mobitz type 2 second-degree block (Fig. 7-5) the P–R interval remains normal but not every atrial impulse is followed by a ventricular contraction. For example, every second or third ventricular beat is missed (or dropped). The heart rate is regularly irregular, i.e. a pattern of irregularity can be identified.

Second-degree block may resolve into first degree block, or deteriorate into complete heart block, or ventricular standstill.

Third-degree (complete) heart block

In third-degree, or complete, block (Fig. 7-6) there is no connection between atrial and ventricular activity, all impulses from the atria being completely blocked. Atrial and ventricular activity continue independently. The SA node continues to function and ventricular activity is controlled from an ectopic focus in the ventricle, which becomes the ventricular pacemaker. Thus P waves and also QRST complexes occur regularly but have no relationship to each other.

In the absence of control from the atria, the ventricular rate (referred to as the idioventricular rate), is normally about 35–45 beats/minute, although the exact rate will depend upon the position of damage within the conductive mechanism. Third-degree heart block is usually associated with reduced cardiac output. It may resolve into second-degree heart block, or deteriorate into ventricular standstill. Ventricular standstill, is when the ventricular focus stops firing completely leaving only atrial activity. This may be transient with spontaneous recovery after a few seconds, known as Stokes–Adams attacks. Unresolved ventricular standstill is associated with loss of cardiac output and is a form of cardiac arrest.

AV block following myocardial infarction may be caused by ischaemia or infarction in the tissues in the conductive pathways. Alternatively, oedema/inflammation surrounding damaged tissue may cause temporary conduction defects, if this affects the conductive pathways.

It may be possible to predict the likelihood of conduction defects arising, by careful location of the myocardial damage on 12-lead ECG recordings. For example, the AV nodal artery is a branch of the right coronary artery, thus occlusion of the right coronary, resulting in inferior infarction, may result in conduction defects, which may be transient in nature. AV block associated with an anterior infarction represents significant myocardial damage and carries a poor prognosis.

NURSING ASSESSMENT

Bradycardia may be detected:

- Coincidentally during the recording of routine observations; in this case, the patient is often asymptomatic, although careful assessment may reveal the presence of associated symptoms.
- By direct observation of a cardiac monitor.
- As a result of responding to symptoms experienced by the patient, or witnessed by the nurse, e.g. feeling dizzy or fainting.

Bradycardia may be sustained, transient or intermittent. Transient bradycardia may last for a few seconds or minutes, or may be present for the duration of an episode causing the bradycardia, e.g. while the patient is vomiting or during endotracheal suctioning.

Transient bradycardias clearly have less sustained effect on cardiac output and may resolve before full assessment can occur. However, the fact that a bradycardia is not sustained does not necessarily mean that it is insignificant. It may indicate a deterioration in the patient's condition, which warrants careful observation since a sustained bradycardia may follow. This is particularly so in patients who may be identified as 'at risk' by nature of the position of their myocardial infarction, or current drug therapy, for example.

The immediate urgency of the situation will depend upon the effect of the bradycardia upon the cardiac output. Assessment must proceed in a logical sequence, in order to ensure that appropriate action is taken in the event of a deterioration in the patient's condition.

Once a bradycardia has been identified, ensure the patient has a patent airway and adequate ventilation. Hypoxia is a cause of bradycardia and obstruction or partial obstruction of the airway must always be considered in semiconscious or unconscious patients. Patients following myocardial infarction are often treated with opiate analgesia and respiratory depression (or respiratory arrest) may occur as a side-effect. If there is any compromise to the airway or respiratory effort, which is not immediately relieved by nursing measures (e.g. suctioning to clear the airway or use of an oral airway to relieve obstruction) resuscitation must be initiated.

Establishing the presence of cardiac output in an unconscious patient can be achieved by palpation of the carotid pulse for a minimum of 5 seconds. This is particularly important in bradycardia, as brief palpation of the pulse may miss the beats completely. Once the presence of cardiac output is established, this can be assessed further by measuring the blood pressure. If this is significantly reduced from the patient's normal range, or abnormally low, immediate medical assistance should be obtained.

If the blood pressure is adequate, the bradycardia should be further assessed. Cardiac monitoring should be initiated, and the bradycardia analysed, to detect the presence of any conduction defect. (Monitoring may reveal the presence of atrial fibrillation, if the bradycardia was caused by a large pulse deficit creating the impression of a radial bradycardia.)

It is useful to obtain a rhythm strip of the bradycardia from the monitor, if facilities allow, for the purposes of analysis and accurate documentation in nursing and/or medical case notes. It may be appropriate for a 12-lead ECG to be recorded during the bradycardia, so that changes in myocardial perfusion may be identified and documented.

If second- or third-degree heart block is detected, the risk of sudden deterioration exists, even if the patient is initially asymptomatic. Assessment of other indices of cardiac output should also be made, e.g. level of consciousness, degree of peripheral perfusion, urine output. While all such observations may be within normal limits initially, they constitute a valuable baseline, should the patient's condition deteriorate.

Other associated symptoms may be present and may provide an indication of the cause of the bradycardia. Pain may indicate myocardial ischaemia, thus the type, location, severity and onset of the pain should be assessed, as well as the need for analgesia. Nausea may be associated with pain, or develop as a side-effect of analgesia or other drug therapies. Nausea may also be associated with gastric engorgement from cardiac failure. It may be helpful to assess the patient's level of activity at the time of onset of the bradycardia, since exertion may precipitate myocardial ischaemia, which in turn may cause a bradycardia. If this is the case, activity levels should be reviewed.

Nursing assessment must be continuous throughout the duration of the bradycardia, as initial tolerance of the reduced heart rate, in terms of maintenance of cardiac output, does not indicate continued tolerance and sudden deterioration may occur at any time.

The intensity of nursing observation will depend upon the overall condition of the patient, the cause of the bradycardia and the actual cardiac rhythm. If the bradycardia is caused by digoxin therapy and the patient has normal cardiac output, nursing observation will be discrete. However, a patient in complete heart block requires constant supervision, since it is a life-threatening dysrhythmia, which may deteriorate into ventricular standstill at any time.

NURSING GOALS

When nursing a patient with bradycardia associated with myocardial infarction, the following nursing goals should be considered:

- Rapid detection of changes in cardiac rhythm and assessment of the impact of the rhythm change on cardiac output.
- Prevention of deterioration in cardiac output, which may extend myocardial damage by increasing myocardial ischaemia.

Rapid detection of changes in cardiac rhythm

Once a bradycardia has been identified and assessed, careful observation is required in order that rhythm changes may be identified promptly and responded to. If a change in cardiac rhythm occurs, complete reassessment is required.

Observation of cardiac rhythm must be accompanied by observation of the rhythm's effect on cardiac output. This may be assessed by monitoring:

- Pulse, blood pressure and right atrial (central venous) pressure (if possible).
- Peripheral perfusion.
- Urine output.
- Level of consciousness.

Effective observation can only be achieved if the following principles are adhered to:

- The patient's bed should be located in an appropriate position in order that both patient and cardiac monitor can be easily seen.
- The availability of resuscitation equipment should also be considered.

Subtle changes in rhythm or condition are most easily recognized by a consistent observer, thus the allocation of one nurse to observe the patient per shift is recommended.

Detailed and accurate communication between nursing staff is essential. The use of rhythm strips for comparative purposes may be helpful.

Accurate documentation of all observations to facilitate the development of 'trends' in the patient's progress is required. Such observations should be carried out as frequently as the patient's condition dictates, while considering the patient's need for rest and sleep. Electronic monitoring equipment, e.g. automatic sphygmomanometers, allows for frequent observation with minimal disruption to the patient.

The patient and any relatives/friends should be informed how to summon nursing assistance, since the patient may develop new symptoms, or visitors witness a sudden deterioration in the patient's condition.

Prevention of deterioration

Deterioration in cardiac output may extend myocardial damage by increasing myocardial ischaemia. It is not always possible to prevent deterioration of cardiac output; however, certain nursing measures may have some effect and, in some cases, will prove successful. Three aspects of care should be considered:

- Reduction of cardiac workload.
- Maximising myocardial oxygenation.
- Avoidance of factors that may precipitate or exacerbate bradycardia.

Reduction in cardiac workload is achieved by resting the patient as completely as possible. Initially bed rest is required, which is maintained for the duration of serious dysrhythmias. Once bed rest is no longer required, gradual remobilisation over a period of days is planned to avoid sudden increases in workload. It should be recognised that some activities require more energy when performed in bed, classically using a bedpan! Commodes are preferable.

Responding to medical staff and visitors also requires effort, so the care of unstable patients should be organised to minimise disruption. Patients find it difficult to rest adequately if constantly disturbed by a stream of visitors who may include nursing staff, nursing students, junior medical staff, senior medical staff, medical students, radiographers, venesectionists, domestic staff, clerical staff, friends and relations!

To achieve adequate rest will require nursing intervention, to ensure that the patient is able to fulfil appropriate activities of living, especially to fulfil individual needs related to mobility, hygiene, elimination, eating and drinking. The importance of excellent psychological care, to minimise patient anxiety and promote adequate rest and relaxation, must not be underestimated.

Myocardial hypoxia is both caused by reduced cardiac output and a cause of reduced cardiac output, since hypoxia exerts a negative inotropic effect on myocardial tissue. It may be caused by myocardial ischaemia or inadequate arterial oxygen saturation; it may also be reduced by reduction in cardiac workload and by drug therapy.

Inadequate arterial saturation may be resolved by ensuring a patent airway and good respiratory effort and by enriching the concentration of inspired oxygen. Oxygen may be administered via face-mask or nasal cannula, the concentration prescribed depending on the result of arterial blood gas analysis.

Some of the causes of bradycardia, and therefore of potential compromise of cardiac output, can be avoided when patients are considered 'at risk'. Most patients following myocardial infarction fall into this category. Straining at stool and vomiting, both of which stimulate the vagus nerve, can be avoided, as can any compromise to the airway and prolonged hypoxia.

Some drug therapy prescribed prior to the development of bradycardia may be inappropriate if a bradycardia develops following myocardial infarction, e.g. digoxin, beta blockers, lignocaine. Such drugs should not be administered and medical staff consulted.

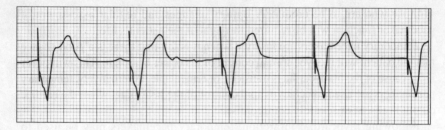

Fig. 7-7 ECG showing paced beats. From Conover, M. B.(1986). *Pocket Nurse Guide to Electrocardiography*, Mosby-Year Book, St Louis, p. 174

The medical management of bradycardia may include drug therapy, e.g. bolus injections of atropine and occasionally isoprenaline infusion, or the use of a temporary cardiac pacemaker.

PACEMAKERS

A cardiac pacemaker is a device that delivers rhythmical electrical impulses to the myocardium, in order to produce ventricular contractions and thereby maintain cardiac output. Some patients suffering with bradycardias will require the insertion of a pacemaker to maintain a normal heart rate.

Pacemakers are programmed to function in either demand or fixed-rate pacing mode. Demand pacing is most commonly used. In demand mode, the pacemaker will only deliver an electrical pulse to stimulate the myocardium when the heart does not generate a beat of its own. The pacemaker is able to 'sense' (or detect) natural beats and these will suppress pacemaker activity. There must be no competition between a paced beat (Fig. 7-7) and a natural beat. If a paced beat competes with a natural beat, there is a risk of the paced QRS complex falling in the vulnerable refractory period of a natural beat, and this can precipitate ventricular fibrillation. (This can also occur with ventricular ectopic beats, the so called 'R on T' phenomena.)

In demand pacing, the rate is set and the pacemaker will cut in and maintain that rate whenever the heart fails to do so. Thus if a demand pacemaker is set at 70 beats/minute and the patient's heart rate is 75 beats/minute the pacemaker will sense this activity and not function. However, if the patient's heart rate falls to 50 beats/minute, the pacemaker will begin to pace at a rate of 70 beats/minute.

In fixed-rate pacing, the pacemaker is set at a given rate and will function at that rate regardless of any natural cardiac activity. This can lead to the possibility of competition between paced and natural beats, as already mentioned.

Temporary and permanent pacemakers

Permanent pacemakers are inserted into the upper chest wall, between the subcutaneous fat and the muscle layer, under local or general anaesthesia. They remain in situ for the rest of the patient's life and should be removed *post mortem* in those who are to be cremated. Battery changes and regular assessment of pacemaker function will be required throughout the patient's life.

Temporary pacemakers are inserted when it is felt that there is a good chance that the patient will recover normal control of his or her heart rate. This will occur if the cause of the bradycardia is transient, or remediable. Alternatively, temporary pacemakers are used to achieve rapid control of the heart rate, when the cardiac output is absent or severely compromised.

Following myocardial infarction, temporary pacemakers may be used to overcome acute dysrhythmias. Few of these patients require permanent pacemakers in the long term.

Indications for temporary pacing

Pacing may be considered in any situation when bradycardia is compromising cardiac output, or when the cardiac output is adequate but deterioration is considered inevitable, for example in:

- Asystole.
- Ventricular standstill.
- Complete heart block.
- Second-degree heart block.
- Stokes–Adams attacks.
- Drug toxicity, either accidental or in deliberate poisoning, with drugs known to cause bradycardia, e.g. digoxin, beta-blockers.

A variety of techniques are available to achieve temporary pacing; these include transoesophageal pacing, transcutaneous (or external) pacing and the transvenous insertion of a temporary pacing wire.

Transoesophageal pacing
The success of transoesophageal pacing is the result of the anatomical proximity of the posterior of the heart to the lower end of the oesophagus.

An oesophageal pacing wire (or electrode) must be used and is inserted into the oesophagus in the same way as a nasogastric tube is passed. If the patient is conscious, intravenous sedation may be helpful. If the patient is unconscious, a laryngoscope may be used to facilitate this process. The position of the wire is adjusted until satisfactory pacing is achieved, as demonstrated by cardiac monitoring. Once in place, the wire is taped into position.

A special pacing box must be used, since transoesophageal pacing requires higher levels of electrical stimulation than transvenous pacing as there is no direct contact with the myocardium.

The great strength of transoesophageal pacing is the speed at which insertion can be achieved, clearly an advantage in immediately life-threatening situations, such as during cardiac arrest. The insertion procedure is straightforward, requiring no particular skill or experience on the part of the medical staff. No particular procedures are required to verify the position of the wire, except to ensure that it is has not been inadvertently passed into the lungs (this is a potential problem in unconscious patients). There are no serious complications and damage to the oesophagus does not appear to occur. Some patients complain of discomfort in the throat. The main disadvantage of this technique is that despite external fixing of the pacing wire, the wire can be mobile in the oesophagus and affected by peristalsis. Consequently, pacing activity may be lost. Specialised transoesophageal pacing equipment must be available and readily accessible in emergencies.

Transcutaneous (external) pacing
Transcutaneous pacing is achieved by passing electrical stimulation to the heart through the chest wall. Large, self adhesive electrodes (similar to ECG electrodes) are attached to the patient – one on the front of the chest and one on the back. The electrodes are pre-gelled with conductive gel and good skin contact is required. The skin should be clean and dry, and free from powder, creams etc. It may be necessary to remove some hair from the chest in order to obtain a good contact. At the same time ECG electrodes are positioned to monitor the patient's cardiac rhythm, to allow for the sensing of natural 'QRS' complexes by the pacemaker, enabling demand pacing to occur. Once positioned, the electrodes are connected to the pacemaker and the level of electrical stimulation adjusted to achieve pacing, while minimising discomfort to the patient. As with transoesophageal pacing, the main strength of transcutaneous pacing is the speed and ease with which it can be initiated – an advantage in emergency situations.

The main disadvantage is the discomfort caused to the patient. Chest pain results from muscular contractions caused by the electrical stimulation, thus analgesia and sedation may be required. If the patient is conscious, careful explanation must be given regarding the procedure and he or she should be warned that discomfort may occur. The degree of patient discomfort must be considered if long-term use of transcutaneous pacing is contemplated.

Transvenous pacing
Transvenous pacing involves the insertion of a pacing wire into the right ventricle of the heart via the venous system. If possible, patient consent should be obtained since this is an invasive procedure. Cardiac monitoring must be maintained throughout the procedure and the position of the chest electrodes may require adjustment.

Before the wire is inserted it is important to check that the pacing box to be used is functioning and that all electrical connections fit together. An aseptic technique is essential and local anaesthesia used. The pacing wire is passed into the right atrium via venepuncture of the right or left subclavian vein (brachial or jugular veins are used occasionally). The wire is then advanced through the tricuspid valve into the right ventricle, the progress of the wire being monitored radiographically using image intensification. Passage of the wire through the tricuspid valve can cause irritation and precipitate ventricular dysrhythmias, careful observation of cardiac rhythm at this stage is therefore essential.

Once the pacing wire is positioned correctly, with the tip of the wire in contact with the endocardium of the right ventricle (Fig. 7-8), the pacemaker can be connected and switched on. The pacing threshold should be established. This is the minimum voltage required to induce ventricular contraction. Initially, a low threshold may be achieved but this may increase in the days following insertion

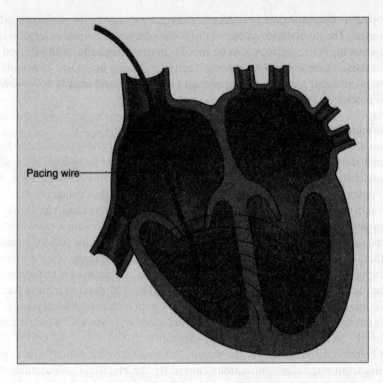

Fig. 7-8 Correct position of the pacing wire in the right ventricle. Adapted from Flynn, J., Bruce, N. (1993). *Introduction to Critical Care Skills*, Mosby-Year Book, St Louis, p.144.

of the pacing wire, since scar tissue forms. Therefore the pacing threshold should be checked daily to ensure that the pacemaker is set at a voltage that will maintain pacing activity. Once the threshold has been established satisfactorily, the wire is sutured in position and a sterile dressing, which allows observation of the insertion site, applied. The procedure is followed by chest X-ray, to verify the position of the pacing wire and to exclude pneumothorax.

The patient's condition is usually improved following the establishment of effective pacing because the cardiac output is increased. However, careful observation of the patient is still required to ensure patient stability.

Care must be taken that the pacing wire is not dislodged, since this will result in a cessation of pacing activity. Patients should be instructed to avoid raising their arms (on the affected side) to above shoulder height. If it is necessary to lift the patient, the shoulder lift (Australian lift) should be avoided if at all possible. Particular care is required if the patient is confused and unable to comply with nursing instructions.

Monitoring of the cardiac output should continue, the frequency of observation being reduced as the patient's condition allows. Gradual mobilisation is permitted with the pacing wire *in situ*, if appropriate.

Careful explanation to the patient and relatives should be given regarding the purpose and functioning of the pacing wire, to reduce anxiety and ensure cooperation. The temporary nature of the pacing wire must be made clear, with the reassurance that a permanent pacemaker is often not required.

A nurse responsible for a patient with a pacing wire *in situ*, must also be responsible for the safety of the pacemaker.

- The pacing wire must be sutured in place and secured with a sterile dressing.
- All connections must be secure and clearly visible, so that disconnection may be detected rapidly.
- The pacing box should be positioned appropriately and be clearly visible at all times.
- The patient must be aware of the need to avoid wire displacement.
- The pacing threshold must be checked every day (either by experienced nursing or medical staff).
- The state of the pacemaker battery must be checked every shift (via battery indicator); replacement batteries must be instantly available.
- Caution should be exercised with other items of electrical equipment (e.g. electric razors, floor polishers etc.) since interference with pacemaker activity may occur.

Complications may arise following the insertion of a temporary pacing wire. These include:

- Pneumothorax and/or internal haemorrhage, usually related to the insertion procedure.
- Infection, either localised at the insertion site, or developing into septicaemia or endocarditis. This may be prevented by the use of a strict aseptic technique at the time of insertion, followed by meticulous wound care. Prophylactic antibiotic therapy may be considered after insertion.
- The pacemaker may fail to initiate a ventricular contraction.

Failure of the pacemaker to initiate ventricular activity, may result from several causes. There may be a loose connection or a disconnection in the pacing circuit. The tip of the pacing wire may have become displaced in the right ventricle so that it is no longer in contact with the endocardium. The pacemaker batteries may have failed, or the pacemaker failed for some other reason. If the pacing wire has become dislodged, this can be detected by observing the ECG. The characteristic pacing 'spike' will be present; however, this is not always followed by a QRS complex. This situation is referred to as 'loss of capture' or 'failure to capture' (Fig. 7-9).

'Delayed capture', when the pacing spike is followed by a QRS complex but not promptly, indicates that there is difficulty in achieving ventricular activity and may precede total loss of capture, alerting the nurse to potential complications. Pacemaker failure (either from disconnection or battery failure) can also be detected on the ECG, as the pacing spike will be absent and the heart rate may fall below the preset rate. The effect on the patient of the failure of a pacemaker to initiate ventricular activity (and thus the urgency of the situation if this occurs), will depend upon the patient's underlying cardiac rhythm and his or her ability to maintain an adequate cardiac output unaided.

Some patients may have reverted to sinus rhythm and be little affected by the pacemaker failure. Others may be able to sustain some cardiac output with a

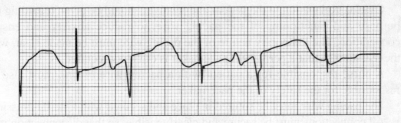

Fig. 7-9 ECG in failure to capture. From Conover, M.B. (1986) *Pocket Nurse Guide to Electrocardiography*, Mosby-Year Book, St Louis, p. 181.

bradycardic rhythm; however, others may become immediately asystolic, with no cardiac output. Urgent action is then required to remedy the situation if possible (e.g. by reconnecting the pacing wire or replacing the battery), while at the same time summoning urgent medical aid and initiating cardiopulmonary resuscitation.

A temporary pacing wire may be removed once the patient's electrical conduction system of the heart has recovered and sinus rhythm is restored. The time taken for this to occur varies from individual to individual; in some cases it may not occur. In this case, a permanent pacemaker is inserted.

Recovery of the patient's conducting system is usually indicated by a gradual reduction in pacing activity, as the heart initiates its own activity. Prior to removal, the pacemaker may be switched off while still *in situ*, to ensure that normal conduction can be maintained.

FURTHER READING

Appel-Hardin, S., Dente-Cassidy, A.M. (1991). How to use a noninvasive temporary pacemaker. *Nursing*, **21(5)**: 58–64.

Conover, M.B. (1994). *Pocket Guide to Electrocardiography*, 3rd edn, Mosby Year Book, St Louis.

Conover, M.B. (1986). *Pocket Nurse Guide: Electrocardiography*, Mosby Year Book, St Louis.

Haught, J. (1993). Catching up with cardiac pacing. *Emergency*, **February**: 4043.

Jowett, N. and Thompson, D. (1989). *Comprehensive Coronary Care*, Scutari Press, London, pp. 286–299.

Mickus, D., Monahan, K., Brown, C. (1986). Exciting external pacemakers. *American Journal of Nursing*, **April**: 403–405.

Strauss McErlean, E., Whitman, G. R. (1991). Therapeutic modalities in the treatment of the patient with cardiovascular dysfunction, in: *Critical Care Nursing: Clinical Management Through the Nursing Process*, Dolan, J. (ed., F. A. Davis Company, Philadelphia.

8.

TACHYCARDIA

The patient who presents with a tachycardia requires careful assessment. Patient outcomes are dependent largely on the ability to recognise and interpret various rhythms and to initiate and/or anticipate the appropriate management response. Any increase in heart rate results in an increase in cardiac muscle work and myocardial oxygen consumption. Tachycardia may be defined as a heart rate above 100 beats/minute in an adult. Types of tachycardia include:

- Sinus tachycardia.
- Paroxysmal atrial tachycardia with or without block.
- Supraventricular tachycardia.
- Junctional or nodal tachycardia.
- Atrial flutter.
- Atrial fibrillation.
- Ventricular tachycardia.
- Ventricular fibrillation.

The causes of tachycardia include:

- Increased physical exertion or effort.
- Strong emotions such as anger, fear, anxiety or stress.
- Pain.
- Shock.
- Cardiac disease.
- Pyrexia sepsis.
- Hypokalaemia.
- Drug effects (e.g. adrenaline, isoprenaline, dopamine, salbutamol).
- Stimulants (e.g. coffee, tea, tobacco).
- Vagal inhibition.
- Hyperthyroidism (excess of circulating thyroxine).

SINUS TACHYCARDIA

In sinus tachycardia the configuration of the PQRST complex and the P–R interval remain normal. The heart rate is regular above 100 beats/minute and may reach 130–140 beats/minute, even at rest. Sinus tachycardia (Fig. 8-1) has many causes, it is a normal physiological response to physical effort, stimulants and stressful or strong emotions or feelings. It can also be associated with heart failure, cardiogenic shock, hypovolaemic shock, myocardial infarction, pulmonary embolism, pericarditis, cardiac tamponade, drug effects or pyrexia. Treatment is directed at the cause. The presence of a sinus tachycardia should alert the nurse to make a full assessment of the patient's condition. There may be some obvious

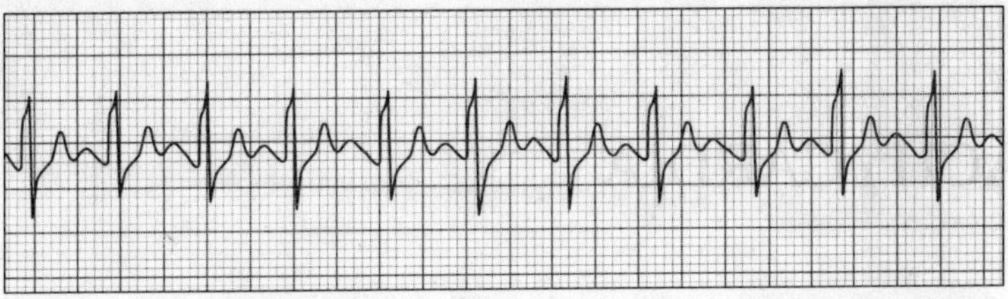

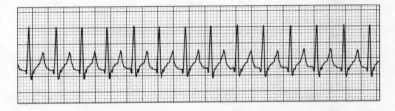

Fig. 8-1 ECG trace showing sinus tachycardia. From Conover, M.B.(1994). *Pocket Guide to Electrocardiography*, Mosby-Year Book, St Louis, p.23.

Fig. 8-2 ECG trace showing atrial tachycardia.

contributing factors that one may have some control over, e.g. the anxious patient or the patient in pain. Alternatively the assessment of cardiac output may indicate a serious deterioration in the patient's condition.

PAROXYSMAL ATRIAL TACHYCARDIA

Atrial tachycardia (Fig. 8-2) originates from an irritable electrical focus in the atria. It is often preceded by atrial ectopic activity, which may be isolated or be a series of ectopics. The rhythm is characterised by runs of three or more consecutive ectopics. The P waves due to the rapid rate may or may not be clearly identified, the QRS complex is normal and similar to that in sinus rhythm. The rhythm is regular and usually between 140–200 beats/minute.

PAROXYSMAL ATRIAL TACHYCARDIA WITH BLOCK

In paroxysmal atrial tachycardia with block (Fig. 8-3) the degree of block may be variable, e.g. 2:1 or 3:1. In this situation, the bundles of His are unable to conduct every atrial impulse. In 2:1 block only every other P wave is followed by a ventricular contraction. The atrial rate may be 200 beats/minute but the ventricular rate is only 100 beats/minute. Atrial tachycardia with block may be a symptom of digoxin toxicity.

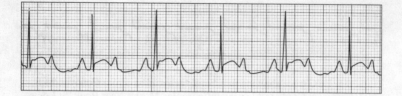

Fig. 8-3 ECG trace showing paroxysmal atrial tachycardia with block. From Conover , M.B. (1994). *Pocket Guide to Electrocardiography*, Mosby-Year Book, St Louis, p.127.

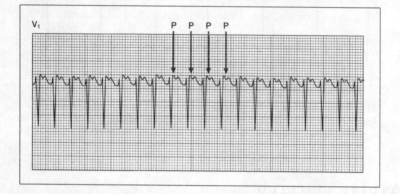

Fig. 8-4 ECG trace showing supraventricular tachycardia. From Conover , M.B. *(1994) Pocket Guide to Electrocardiography*, Mosby-Year Book, St Louis, p.66.

SUPRAVENTRICULAR TACHYCARDIA

As the name would suggest, this rhythm (Fig. 8-4) originates above the bifurcation of the bundle of His. The term 'supraventricular' is used frequently when it is impossible to see the P waves, which may be hidden in the preceding T wave. The QRS complex is normal but may be narrowed in appearance. This rapid regular rhythm can vary between 150–250 beats/minute. It may occur in short bursts, when it is termed paroxysmal. This rhythm can occur in the healthy heart or in patients suffering from cardiac disease. It is also associated with Wolf-Parkinson-White syndrome.

JUNCTIONAL TACHYCARDIA

Impulses originate from an area surrounding the AV node. These impulses are conducted normally through the ventricles. Inverted P waves with a short PR interval may be identified (Fig.8–5). Alternatively, P waves may be lost completely within the QRS complex. This feature is due to the extremely short time lapse between atrial and ventricular excitation. Occasionally the P waves may be seen after the QRS complex. The rate is usually between 140–200 beats per minute.

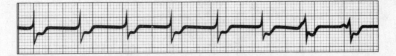

Fig. 8-5 ECG trace showing junctional tachycardia. From Conover, M.B. *(1994). Pocket Guide to Electrocardiography*, Mosby-Year Book, St Louis, p.23.

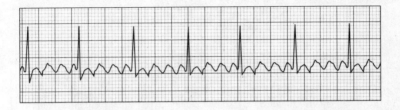

Fig. 8-6 ECG trace showing atrial flutter. From Conover, M.B. *Pocket Guide to Electrocardiography*, Mosby-Year Book, St Louis, p.48.

ATRIAL FLUTTER

In this rhythm (Fig. 8-6), rapid regular atrial excitation occurs. It is termed 'flutter' as the very rapid P waves have a characteristic saw-tooth appearance and are usually called 'F' waves. These rapid atrial deflections can occur at a rate of 240–360/minute. The ventricles cannot respond to every F wave, so there is always a degree of physiological block. The degree of block may be variable such that the QRS complex may occur regularly or irregularly. The ventricular rate may be between 120–180 beats/minute, depending on the degree of block. This rhythm usually occurs in the abnormal heart, it is possible for flutter to precede atrial fibrillation. Atrial flutter is seen in patients with progressive heart failure, particularly those with mitral valve disease.

ATRIAL FIBRILLATION

This rhythm is characteristically an irregular rhythm of variable rate. The term fibrillation describes the uncoordinated twitching movement of the atria, resulting in bizarre atrial deflections, which are rapid and chaotic. There is no discrete atrial contraction and relaxation so that the atrial contribution to cardiac output is lost.

The rate of ventricular response is variable. Atrial activity may be 300–600 beats/minute. Some of these impulses enter theAV node and generate irregular QRS complexes at varying rates, depending on conduction. Fast atrial fibrillation may present at a rate of 150 beats/minute or more. In slow atrial fibrillation, the ventricular rate can be as slow as 50 beats/minute. Patients in atrial fibrillation should have their heart rate counted for at least 30 seconds.

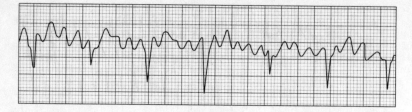

Fig. 8-7 ECG traces showing fine atrial fibrillation with uncontrolled ventricular response. From Conover, M.B. *Pocket Guide to Electrocardiography*, Mosby-Year Book, St Louis, p.53.

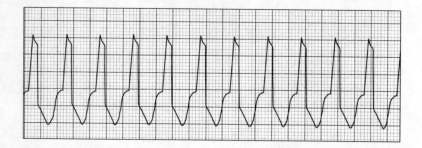

Fig. 8-8 ECG trace showing ventricular tachycardia. From Conover, M.B. *Pocket Guide to Electrocardiography*, Mosby-Year Book, St Louis, p.23.

Observation of the apex and pulse rate simultaneously will identify the rate differential. Atrial fibrillation (Fig. 8-7) can be chronic, acute or paroxysmal. It is associated with enlarged atria and is frequently present in patients with mitral valve disease. It may also be present in ischaemic heart disease following myocardial infarction, congestive heart failure, pulmonary embolism and thyrotoxicosis.

RHYTHM DISTURBANCES ARISING IN THE VENTRICLES

All tachycardias are potentially serious and may lead to further clinical deterioration; however, ventricular dysrhythmias are life-threatening and will rapidly, if not immediately, potentiate a loss of consciousness and cardiac arrest.

Ventricular tachycardia

This rhythm originates from an irritable focus in the ventricle and may be preceded by ventricular ectopic activity. Three or more consecutive ventricular ectopic beats constitute a ventricular tachycardia. Alternatively, it may be sustained or convert into ventricular fibrillation.

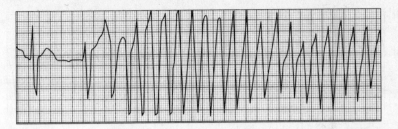

Fig. 8-9 ECG trace showing ventricular fibrillation. From Conover, M.B. (1994) *Pocket Guide to Electrocardiography*, Mosby-Year Book, St Louis, p.93.

Ventricular tachycardia (Fig. 8-8) is usually a regular rhythm with a rate of 140–200 beats/minute. The QRS complexes are broad and there is rarely any evidence of atrial activity. This does not indicate absence of atrial activity but relates to the rapid discharge rate of the ventricular ectopic focus, which becomes the dominant one. Occasionally, a P wave may be visible but it bears no relationship to the QRS complex, unless it is a 'capture' beat. In this instance, a normal sinus complex appears. Absence of synchronised atrial activity and the accompanying inefficient ventricular contraction that occurs in this rhythm will result in a dramatic drop or loss of blood pressure. Ventricular tachycardia occurs in severe heart disease, e.g. following acute myocardial infarction. It can be precipitated by hypokalaemia, severe hypoxia and/or acidosis and hypotension.

There are instances when an episode of ventricular tachycardia is well tolerated in terms of its effect on the circulation, level of consciousness and cardiac output. These episodes may self-terminate spontaneously. If appropriate, requesting the patient to cough, or administering a precordial thump to the chest can occasionally stimulate a return to the patient's normal rhythm.

Ventricular fibrillation

In ventricular fibrillation (Fig. 8-9) there is no coordinated activity of the ventricles. The only signs of electrical activity are irregular waves of varying sizes that have no evidence of PQRST waveforms. These waves may occur at a rate of 300–500 beats/minute. There is no effective pumping action and no adequate cardiac output. Cardiopulmonary resuscitation will be necessary immediately. As in ventricular tachycardia, this rhythm is associated with severe heart disease, particularly acute myocardial infarction.

NURSING ASSESSMENT

Identifying the presence of a tachycardia may occur in the following ways:

- Direct observation of the monitored ECG.
- During the course of routine observation or the giving of care.
- The patient informing the nurse of symptoms associated with the rhythm change or as a result of the change.
- By the nurse observing and assessing various degrees of deterioration in a patient's condition.

The tachycardia may occur intermittently, i.e. be paroxysmal, transient or sustained. The dysrhythmia may be initiated by a specific event such as effort, over-exertion or stimulants, or as a side-effect of other therapy, i.e. drugs that may increase heart rate, salbutamol, adrenaline, high doses of dopamine or dobutamine. Alternatively, the tachycardia may occur while the patient is at rest. Episodes of tachycardia are significant as they may indicate a change in the patient's condition or may become sustained.

At the onset of a tachycardia, the patient may well become aware of a sudden increase, irregularity or change in force of their heart rate. They may complain of a sensation of fluttering or palpitations in their chest and alert nurses accordingly. This is frequently a very unpleasant and potentially frightening experience, particularly if accompanied by feeling breathless, dizzy or light-headed. Increasing anxiety may further compound the problem. The assessment needs to be conducted in an efficient and reassuring manner, the urgency and speed of assessment will be dictated by the immediately observed effects on the patient's cardiac output.

It is of importance to remember that certain warning signs, i.e. atrial or ventricular ectopic activity may precede a tachycardia. In the patient whose ECG is not being monitored continuously, this type of activity may be detected by noting dropped beats, irregular beats or spurts of rapid or absent pulse rate when taking a pulse. A 12-lead ECG will be essential to diagnose correctly the rhythm and potentially facilitate treatment that will prevent more serious rhythm disturbances occurring.

In the monitored patient, ectopic activity requires careful observation for frequency, pattern and effect of occurrence. Obtaining a rhythm strip will aid further assessment. In some patients, mild ectopic activity is well tolerated and acceptable. However, medical staff should be informed if it is a new event, if runs of ectopics occur, there is a change in the pattern of occurrence or an increase in the number of ectopic beats over a minute. Criteria will need to be identified and agreed with medical staff in respect of the reporting and management of any changes.

A form of ventricular ectopic activity that may frequently lead to ventricular tachycardia or fibrillation is the 'R on T' phenomenon, that is, if the R wave of the ectopic beat falls near the peak of the T wave of the preceding beat. Atrial or ventricular ectopic activity may be precipitated by a low serum potassium. Treatment should be aimed at maintaining serum potassium levels at 4–4.5 mmol/litre.

ASSESSMENT OF THE TACHYCARDIC PATIENT

Once it has been determined that the patient is tachycardic, it is essential to undertake a swift comprehensive assessment of the patient's condition and physical tolerance of the rhythm. This assessment must include the following, and is particularly relevant in the presence of ventricular rhythm disturbances.

- Determine the level of consciousness.
- Ensure the patient has an unobstructed airway and adequate ventilation.
- Establish the presence of cardiac output by palpation of the carotid pulse for a minimum of 5 seconds.

If the patient is in cardiac and or respiratory arrest, commence resuscitation procedures immediately and send for urgent medical aid. If the patient is tachycardic with a cardiac output and has adequate ventilation, medical staff should be informed and the assessment should proceed as follows and medical staff should be informed.

- *Measure the blood pressure.* If the blood pressure is adequate, monitoring of the ECG should be commenced. This will enable the tachycardia to be analysed and myocardial perfusion to be assessed. A significant drop in blood pressure or a systolic pressure of less than 100 mmHg may well indicate a change in haemodynamic status caused by the tachycardia, e.g. rapid atrial fibrillation precipitating a subsequent drop in blood pressure. Alternatively, the tachycardia may be a response to a low blood pressure (e.g. a patient may be in shock following myocardial infarction or haemorrhage); this is usually a sinus tachycardia. The increase in heart rate is a physiological response in an effort to maintain cardiac output.
- *Monitor the rate and depth of respiration.* The patient should be observed for signs of increasing respiratory effort and/or cyanosis, which may be caused by pulmonary oedema as a result of a cardiac failure or hypoxia. The administering of oxygen by face mask may be necessary or beneficial to the patient's comfort and ease of ventilation.
- *Assess the level of consciousness.* This may vary in different situations, relating to cardiac output and oxygenation and subsequent effect on cerebral perfusion.
- *Assess the skin turgidity and peripheral perfusion.* The skin may be pale and sweaty, extremities may be cold and poorly perfused as a result of reduced cardiac output.
- *Assess pain.* The patient in pain may well be tachycardic. In the case of chest pain, this may indicate an episode of acute angina or myocardial infarction with accompanying rapid rhythm disturbance. The need for analgesia and/or further action should therefore be assessed.
- *Measure central venous pressure* (if possible). A drop in venous pressure may indicate hypovolaemic shock, whereas an elevated venous pressure may indicate a degree of heart failure. Either may be accompanied by a drop in blood pressure.
- *Measure the patient's temperature.* The presence of a pyrexia may indicate a septic patient.
- *Monitor urine output.* This will diminish rapidly in the presence of a low cardiac output. An inadequate urine output will embarrass further the failing heart.

Careful assessment of these parameters will give a clearer picture of the presenting condition and provide a baseline for reassessment should the patient's condition deteriorate further. Alterations or abnormal parameters will necessitate obtaining medical advice and assistance. Obtaining a rhythm strip or 12-lead ECG, and ensuring that the patient's observations and conditions are recorded clearly will provide a comprehensive documentation of the event. It is possible that initial assessment may indicate little or no deterioration in the patient's condition. Any subsequent changes may be insidious or of acute onset. In several instances, a decision will be made to treat the rhythm before any further deterioration occurs, it is for this reason that medical staff should be informed.

GOALS OF CARE

When nursing a patient with a tachycardia, the following nursing goals should be considered:

- Rapid detection of a change in cardiac rhythm and its impact on cardiac output.
- The prevention of any further deterioration in cardiac output.

Following the initial event, patients will require careful reassessment and monitoring at regular intervals. The extent to which they are monitored and observed will depend largely on the seriousness and stability of their condition and their response to treatment. Frequent observation may, on occasion, be tiring and anxiety-provoking for the patient. The use of electrical monitoring equipment for ECG and blood pressure limits the need for disturbance, allowing vital periods of rest.

One important consideration is the location of the patient's bed, which should readily facilitate the level of observation necessary. The unstable, monitored patient should be in a position where both the patient and monitor are easily seen and quickly accessed. Resuscitation equipment should also be positioned conveniently.

The nurse allocated to the care of the unstable patient will need to be competent in the necessary assessment and evaluation skills. The recommendation of one such nurse per shift is valuable for a variety of reasons. Subtle changes in rhythm or condition are often observed more readily by a consistent observer. Providing continuity of care will also help promote a therapeutic relationship between the nurse, patient and family. The anticipation and experience of a sudden rhythm change can create anxieties, such that the nurse clearly has a role in assessing and, where possible, allaying any fears the patient and family may have. To an extent this is achieved by ensuring information needs and coping strategies are identified, met and supported as much as possible.

THE PREVENTION OF ANY FURTHER DETERIORATION IN CARDIAC OUTPUT

In the process of caring for a patient who is tachycardic or has an unstable rhythm, certain nursing considerations may prevent a further deterioration in cardiac output. Important factors influencing care will include:

- Any potential impact or affect on cardiac output.
- Potential impact or affect on oxygenation and myocardial perfusion
- Situations that may precipitate or exacerbate a tachycardia.

The degree of activity and or mobility in which the patient engages requires careful assessment in relation to these considerations.

During the acute period, the provision of adequate rest and sleep periods will be essential in order to optimise cardiac output and oxygenation. Nursing observation and care should be organised to promote this as much as possible. This consideration will frequently need extending to other staff and those members of the multidisciplinary team who may visit or attend to the patient. Identifying specific rest periods for patients or ensuring whenever possible they are not disturbed when asleep will promote this and be beneficial. The patient may gain considerable comfort and reassurance from visits from family and close friends; however, there is the risk that large numbers of, or frequent visitors may be quite exhausting. This situation requires tact and discussion with the family. Decisions regarding visiting should be made on the basis of what is right for an individual patient and family unit where possible, and evaluated as necessary.

Excellent psychological care and information-giving can contribute enormously to the reassurance of patient and family. This will include clear and concise treatment and progress reports from medical and nursing staff as and when appropriate.

As the patient's condition improves, activity and mobilisation can increase. This will require careful supervision and observation initially, to ensure that it is not 'too much, too soon' in terms of exertion and effort. This may provoke a subsequent physiological demand, causing a reduction in cardiac output and oxygenation. The provision of adequate oxygenation is noted by careful assessment of respiratory status, as described earlier. The exchange and or transport of oxygen may be affected in the cardiac patient. Additional oxygen administered by face mask or nasal cannula may be required on a continuous or intermittent basis. This requirement for oxygen may relate to the extent any effort or exertion is tolerated by the patient, e.g. the patient may benefit from oxygen when getting out of bed to use a commode.

A variety of situations or factors may precipitate a tachycardic event. A change in cardiac output may precipitate a change in rhythm, just as a change in rhythm may affect cardiac output. Therefore any sudden additional demand in physical or psychological effort or exertion may predispose a change in heart rate and or rhythm.

An individual assessment and awareness of a patient's response or adaptation to any demand is necessary. This assessment should be documented clearly and communicated verbally to other relevant members of staff and care should be planned and delivered accordingly. Any drugs prescribed that may precipitate a tachycardia should not be given and medical staff consulted. The importance of maintaining serum potassium at normal levels has been discussed earlier in this chapter. Abnormal results should be reported promptly to the medical staff so that any necessary treatment can be prescribed.

TREATMENT

The medical management of tachycardia may include a variety of responses, depending on the rhythm, how well it is tolerated and whether it is an acute or chronic episode. Treatments may include the following:

• For an acute episode:
  Treating the cause.
  Carotid sinus massage.
  Cardioversion.
  Defibrillation.
  Drug therapy.
• For a chronic episode:
  Implantable cardioverter defibrillators.
  Intraoperative mapping and endocardial resection.

Treatment for tachycardia will depend on the type of presenting rhythm. Patients may frequently be very anxious during periods of rapid heart rate. This anxiety is often heightened by the activity of nursing and medical staff and the frequent very unpleasant sensation of a pounding rapid heart rate. This uncertainty and anxiety can often compound the situation and cause further acceleration in heart rate. It is important to reassure the patient as much as possible and give careful explanations of what is happening or going to happen.

Treating the cause

This relates predominantly to sinus tachycardia, which may be a symptom of a condition. If it is not a symptom of a correctable psychological or physiological stressor, treatment with a beta-blocker preparation, e.g. propranolol, may be prescribed, provided that the blood pressure is adequate.

Carotid sinus massage

This is a noninvasive method of stimulating the vagus nerve. The carotid sinus is a small widening of the internal carotid artery just above where it branches from the common carotid artery. The wall of the carotid artery contains baroreceptors, which sense any stretch in the artery wall that occurs with an increase in blood pressure. Gentle carotid sinus massage stimulates this effect. Impulses from the baroreceptors are received in the medulla and consequently the cardioinhibitory centre is stimulated and the cardioacceleratory centre is inhibited. Arising from the cardioinhibitory centre are parasympathetic fibres that reach the heart via the vagus nerve. Parasympathetic stimulation will decrease the heart rate. Gentle carotid sinus massage is performed for 10–20 seconds, occasionally this vagal stimulation may produce ventricular ectopic activity, which may be isolated or in short bursts. Therefore, resuscitation equipment should be available. The patient should be nursed in a comfortable position, with their head well supported. Carotid sinus massage should be performed by a member of the medical staff. This method of vagal stimulation may be successful in the management of atrial or supraventricular tachycardia by slowing the ventricular rate. A slower ventricular rate may aid identification of the presence or position of the P waves, carotid sinus massage may restore the patient to normal sinus rhythm.

Synchronised cardioversion

Cardioversion is frequently performed for atrial arrhythmias, when drug or other therapies have failed to return the heart to normal sinus rhythm, or to slow the heart rate effectively. It may also be used if the rhythm is severely affecting cardiac output.

A defibrillator is a standard piece of emergency equipment on hospital wards. It is the responsibility of nursing staff to ensure that it is always in good working order and ready for use. The defibrillator should always be plugged in and charged. Any equipment check should include testing, charging and discharging capacity.

Cardioversion involves delivering an electric shock to the heart. It differs from defibrillation in that the shock is synchronised and triggered by the R wave of the ECG. When a patient is to be cardioverted, it is vital to check that the machine is set to the synchronised mode. The synchronised shock ensures that it does not occur in the vulnerable phase (Fig. 8-10) of the ECG complex, when it could trigger ventricular fibrillation or ventricular tachycardia. The pulse is timed to occur just after the R wave when the myocardial cells are completely refractory.

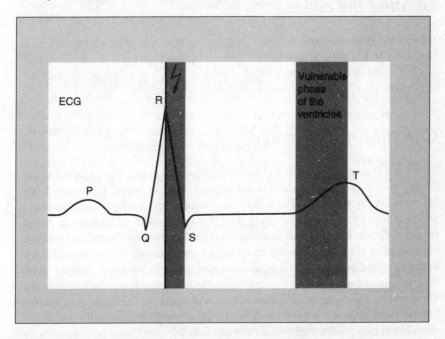

Fig. 8-10 ECG trace showing the vulnerable phase of the ventricles during cardioversion. Adapted from Van der Mosel, H. (1994) *Principles of Biomedical Engineering for Nursing Staff*, Blackwell Scientific, Oxford, p.137.

There has been debate over the safety of cardioversion when patients are digitalised. Cardioversion is not performed in cases of digitalis toxicity, moreover digoxin treatment may be stopped the day before elective cardioversion. Cardioversion may be performed electively or as an emergency intervention.

Preparing the patient for elective cardioversion

Patients may be admitted to hospital for elective cardioversion, or it may be a planned elective procedure during their hospital stay. These patients are usually awake and alert, they should have the procedure explained to them and their consent obtained. They need to be reassured that they will be anaesthetised and not feel the shock. Prior to the anaesthetic they will need to have nothing by mouth for 4–6 hours. In several instances, medical staff may want to be assured that patients in atrial fibrillation are adequately anticoagulated prior to cardioversion. This is a precautionary measure to reduce any risk of a thromboembolic episode occurring. Elective cardioversion is usually performed in the theatre or a room suitable for this procedure.

Preparing the patient for urgent cardioversion

In these instances, the choice to perform the procedure urgently is most likely to be due to the fact that the rhythm is not being well tolerated by the patient. The procedure may be carried out in the ward area. If this is the case, full resuscitation equipment must be readily available. The patient should be informed and reassured as much as is possible. An anaesthetist will be available for this procedure, since it is usual for the patient to sedated and possibly intubated and ventilated in order to protect the airway. The ECG will be monitored continuously. It is of value to obtain a rhythm strip prior to and following the event.

Preparing the patient for cardioversion in the ward area

It is possible that respiration may be depressed or compromised following the administration of sedative drugs, therefore full resuscitation equipment must be readily available. This will include intubation equipment, suction and a means of ventilating the patient. The skin that comes into contact with the defibrillator paddles will need protecting from burns (which can be quite severe). Either the paddles need a thin even layer of electrode gel or, alternatively, the gel pads now available and designed for this purpose should be placed on the patient's chest in the appropriate positions. The paddles are used to deliver the shock. One paddle is placed at the second intercostal space to the right of the sternum. The other paddle is placed over the apex of the heart at the fifth intercostal space to the left of the sternum.

Additional safety considerations

These are as follows:

- Ensure the defibrillator is charged to the appropriate number of Joules requested by the attending physician, e.g. 100 Joules.
- Immediately prior to delivering the shock to the patient, the operator must ensure that everyone, including him- or herself, are standing well clear of the patient's bed, otherwise they may receive part of the shock!

Nursing considerations following cardioversion

Following cardioversion, the patient will require close observation of level of consciousness, also of respiratory and cardiovascular function. There may well be a requirement for oxygen therapy for a period of time, particularly if they are still drowsy. The patient's heart rate, rhythm and blood pressure will require monitoring for any change on a regular basis. There is always the possibility that the rhythm may revert back to the original presenting rhythm.

Emergency defibrillation

Patients in ventricular tachycardia with little or no cardiac output, or ventricular fibrillation will require immediate cardiopulmonary resuscitation and urgent emergency defibrillation. Following emergency defibrillation the probability of a return to automaticity is largely dependent on the duration of these dysrythmias, the metabolic state of the myocardium and the oxygenation of the myocardium. The outcome is therefore significantly improved if defibrillation is prompt (Hendley, 1992). If an initial precardial thump is unsuccessful in ventriclar fibrillation or pulseless ventricular tachycardia this should be followed by a sequence of up to 2 DC shocks of 200 Joules. If these shocks are unsuccessful, a third shock of 360 Joules is administered and resuscitation continued according to European Resuscitation Council and Resuscitation Council UK guidelines.

It is for this reason that, in certain departments and wards, nurses have received specialised training and assessment in the technique of defibrillation enabling them to act promptly and defibrillate in emergency situations. If a suitably trained nurse is not available, valuable time can be saved by ensuring the defibrillator is at the patient's bedside, plugged in and charged to 200 Joules, also that gel pads are readily available to put onto the patient's chest. There is frequently a hive of activity during resuscitation situations. Clear and calm directions need to be given by the most senior nurse available. It is essential that all staff ensure that a safe environment is maintained at all times, in terms of equipment and safety of the other patients.

Nursing considerations following emergency defibrillation

Once the patient has been stabilised, a decision must be made as to whether the patient requires transfer to a high-dependency/intensive care unit, or they can be safely nursed where they are. This will depend largely on their condition and the level of further observation or intervention required. Following resuscitation, patients may remember fragments of events. They may wish to discuss this and they should be given the opportunity to do so, as and when they wish.

Drug therapy

A variety of drugs may be used to control atrial tachycardia. They may be used as a first- or second-line management response depending on the rhythm and effect on cardiac output. These drugs may include digoxin, verapamil, amiodarone and the relatively new drug adenosine for the treatment of supraventricular tachycardia.

Nursing considerations
Patients will require careful monitoring of the effects of the drug on heart rate and rhythm and cardiac output. It is also important to be aware of any side-effects that may occur. Patients who are selected for the following treatments for recurrent ventricular dysrhythmias will be referred to specialised cardiac centres.

Implantable cardiovertor defibrillators

Patients who suffer episodes of recurrent ventricular tachycardia or ventricular fibrillation, in whom management with dysrhythmic drugs has failed. This will not include patients with these dysrhythmias following a *recent* myocardial infarction.

Assessment
This will include electrophysiology studies, testing of exercise tolerance and cardiac catheterisation. An assessment should also be made of the patient's psychological state in terms of coping with device and compliance with follow-up regimens. This implantable device consists of a battery-operated pulse generator and varying lead (or leads).

Insertion technique
This technique may vary from centre to centre. The most recent technique is a transvenous puncture. Usually the subclavian vein is accessed to insert the lead or leads combination. A small incision may also be made at the site of the lead entry in order to insert the cardioverter defibrillator. In some patients, the box may be placed in different positions, e.g. under the rectus sheath. The generator weighs approximately 130–200 g. One lead is always placed in the right ventricle position, whereas the position of the other electrode is variable according to each individual patient. This device is designed to identify the very abnormal QRS complexes associated with ventricular tachycardia/fibrillation. When these dysrhythmias are detected, the device charges and delivers a shock up to 34 Joules. If the first shock fails to terminate the rhythm, the device is programmed to repeat the shock up to four or five times. If these shocks are unsuccessful, resuscitation/external counter shock will be necessary. Implantable cardioverter defibrillators are very sophisticated devices; they can also be programmed to detect a bradycardia and demand pace, or detect a tachycardia and overdrive pace at a faster rate.

Potential complications may include infection, dislodgement of the leads and subclavian vein thrombosis.

Nursing considerations
When caring for a patient with this device, it is essential to know if the device is in the active or deactive mode. If a counter shock is necessary when in the active mode, if the position of the box is known, or can be seen, it is essential to ensure that the defibrillator paddles are at least 25 cm from the box. Patient and family education and support is essential prior to and following insertion of an implantable cardioverter defibrillator.

Intraoperative mapping and endocardial resection

This is a surgical technique for the treatment of ventricular tachycardia when pharmacological preparations appear to be unsuccessful. It is not performed following **recent** myocardial infarction.

Surgical approach
This is via a median sternotomy incision. Simply described, mapping involves programmed electrical stimulation to the epicardial surface of the heart to stimulate ventricular tachycardia. Multiple bipolar electrodes are placed over the heart; computer regeneration of the propagation of the ventricular tachycardia then allows the identification of the origin and its subsequent resection. Following the identification of areas with abnormal electrical foci, the patient is put on cardiopulmonary bypass. The surgeon then resects that area of endocardium and any concomitant procedures, e.g. coronary artery bypass grafting, are performed.

Prior to discharge, thorough assessment of the patient for the occurrence of potential dysrhythmias is important in order to evaluate the success of the surgery.

FURTHER READING

Boltz, M. (1994). Nurses guide to identifying cardiac rhythmns. *Nursing,* **24**: 54–58.

Conover, M.B. (1994). *Pocket Guide to Electrocardiography* (3rd edn.), Mosby Year Book Inc., Missouri.

Flanders, A. (1994). A detailed explanation of defibrillation. *Nursing Times,* **90**: (18) 3739.

Handley, J. (1994). Guidelines for advanced life support: European Resuscitation Council Guidelines. *Resuscitation* **23** (2): 111–122.

Summers, C., O'Mara, R. (1985). Assessment and treatment of life-threatening ventricular arrythmias: The role of programmed electrical stimulation, intraoperative mapping and endocardial resection. *Heart and Lung,* **14** (2): 130–141.

9.

LEFT VENTRICULAR FAILURE AND ACUTE PULMONARY OEDEMA

Left ventricular failure (LVF) is a frequent complication of myocardial infarction and, if severe or refractory to treatment, often indicates a poor prognosis. The onset is often insidious, requiring diligent nursing observation to ensure it is detected rapidly, so that prompt medical treatment may be initiated. Pulmonary oedema is the distressing symptom that occurs in LVF, although it must be remembered that this is not the only cause. Noncardiac causes of pulmonary oedema include exposure to high altitudes, the inhalation of toxic substances, such as chlorine, or following severe head injury or other intracerebral catastrophe. However, this chapter is concerned with cardiac causes, primarily LVF following myocardial infarction.

CARDIAC CAUSES OF LVF

While direct damage to the left ventricle, such as occurs following infarction, is the commonest cause encountered in nursing practice, it may also result from any condition that puts an undue burden on the left ventricle. Thus it may occur as a result of arterial hypertension, cardiomyopathy, or valvular disorders (particularly the aortic and mitral valves). It may also be precipitated in a tachydysrhythmia from inadequate diastolic filling time. In the elderly it may be the first indication of a silent myocardial infarction.

From a physiological point of view, the heart may be considered as forming two separate, but closely related, pumping systems. The right side provides the pump to maintain the pulmonary circulation, while the left side provides the pump for the rest of the body. Thus the right side can afford to operate at lower pressures than the left side. Following myocardial infarction, the damaged areas of the left ventricle are unable to contract normally, thus the pumping ability of the left ventricle is reduced. This leads to a reduction in the stroke volume and ultimately of cardiac output. This reduction in performance means that the left ventricle is unable to empty fully after each contraction and cannot cope with the amount of blood it receives from the pulmonary circulation. Consequently an excess amount of blood remains in the left ventricle after systole. This residual volume gradually increases as the right side of the heart continues to pump normally, which causes a rise in left ventricular diastolic pressure, causing pressure in the left atrium to increase since it can no longer empty completely into the left ventricle. Eventually this increase in pressure is transmitted back along the pulmonary veins to the pulmonary capillaries. This backward transmission of pressure eventually causes fluid to seep into the alveoli, causing pulmonary oedema.

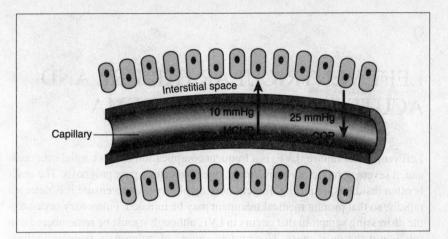

Fig. 9-1 Summary of forces involved in fluid exchange.

Pulmonary oedema is best understood in terms of the mechanisms involved in fluid exchange produced by the pulmonary and systemic circulations (Fig. 9-1). The colloid osmotic pressure (COP) is the pressure produced by the plasma proteins, which tends to draw fluid back into the capillaries and normally measures approximately 25–30 mmHg. Conversely, the mean capillary hydrostatic pressure (MCHP) is the pressure exerted by the blood in the capillaries, which forces fluid out into the interstitial space. The normal MCHP is approximately 15 mmHg. Thus in normal health there is a net difference of 10–15 mmHg, which ensures that more fluid remains in the capillaries than in the interstitial space.

Thus should either the COP decrease (as in a reduction of plasma proteins) or the MCHP increase (as in LVF) there would be a disruption to the normal pressure differences, so allowing more fluid to shift from the capillaries into the interstitial space. This accumulation of fluid in the interstitial space is known as interstitial oedema and is the early manifestation of pulmonary oedema. As such it is symptomless and cannot be detected by physical examination, such as auscultation. It is, however, revealed on chest X-ray (Fig. 9-2) and explains why chest X-rays form one of the most important investigations in coronary care. Eventually as the left ventricular failure progresses, fluid seeps from the interstitial space into the alveoli, producing the characteristic signs and symptoms of overt left ventricular failure.

CONSEQUENCES OF PULMONARY OEDEMA

The accumulation of fluid in the alveoli causes a reduction in pO_2 and an increase in pCO_2. This, coupled with the bronchiole irritation, leads to dyspnoea and tachycardia, since the body tries to compensate and the sympathetic nervous system is activated, producing the characteristic cold, clammy appearance and reflex

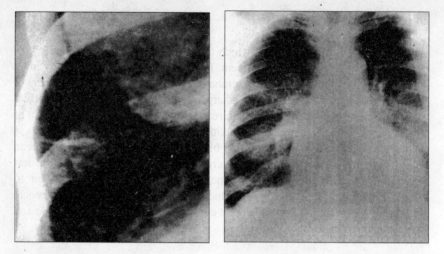

Fig. 9-2 Chest X-rays demonstrating early (left) and late (right) pulmonary oedema. From Conway, N. (1977). *An Atlas of Cardiology*, Wolfe, London, p.8.

peripheral vasoconstriction. The resulting return of deoxygenated blood to the heart is known as shunting and is an example of a ventilation/perfusion mismatch. In severe cases, pulmonary oedema is evidenced by severe dyspnoea and the appearance of pink, frothy fluid so that, effectively, the individual is drowning in their own secretions, thus prompt airway management may be required.

Clinical features

Typically acute pulmonary oedema occurs in the night or early hours of the morning. This is thought to result from the increase in venous return that occurs when lying down. This increases right ventricular output, thus presenting the left ventricle with an extra burden that it is unable to cope with. This produces the usual picture of:

- Sudden onset of moderate to severe dyspnoea.
- A feeling of suffocation accompanied by extreme fear and panic.
- Cold, moist skin and a grey colour.
- Cyanotic nail beds.
- Weak, rapid pulse.
- Distension of neck veins.
- Altered/obtunded mental state.

Medical management

Obviously the clinical setting in which the patients with LVF find themselves will influence the urgency of treatment. For instance, in a patient already in an intensive care environment, who is intubated and ventilated, the development of LVF does not present such a clinical emergency as someone on a general medical ward. Whatever the setting, the initial treatment of LVF and the management of pulmonary oedema is pharmacological in nature. The aim of this treatment is to achieve a reduction in the circulating blood volume, thus reducing the mean capillary hydrostatic pressure and therefore reducing the strain on the left ventricle. Once treatment has commenced, attention should be given to establishing the cause of the problem and hopefully preventing a reoccurrence. In acute LVF, the mainstay of treatment consists of diamorphine, frusemide and oxygen administration.

Diamorphine therapy

Diamorphine is given with care intravenously to reduce the anxiety and so reduce catecholamine secretion. It also produces a degree of peripheral vasodilation, which reduces cardiac afterload. However, because diamorphine is a respiratory depressant, an opiate antagonist (e.g. naloxone) must always be available.

Diuretic therapy

The diuretic of choice is usually frusemide because of its rapid onset of action. It produces symptomatic relief even before the diuresis is evident. Again given intravenously, it causes a fall in blood volume and has a vasodilating effect. Unfortunately it causes the loss of potassium in the urine, so care should be taken that potassium levels do not fall, precipitating dysrhythmias, e.g. ventricular fibrillation.

Oxygen therapy

Oxygen should be given via a face mask in a concentration adequate to counteract the hypoxia. In general, a concentration of 40–60% is necessary, unless there are contraindications, such as chronic lung disease. Ideally it should be monitored by arterial blood gas estimation and transcutaneous oximetry.

Inotropic support/vasodilator therapy

In severe cases, particularly following infarction, inotropic agents (e.g. dobutamine) may be required to assist the left ventricle by increasing myocardial contractility. There is the danger, however, of increasing infarct size from the increase in myocardial oxygen demand caused by these drugs. Similarly, this may predispose to dysrhythmias, so close monitoring is required.

Venesection

This is an older form of treatment, although sometimes still of some use. The withdrawal of 500 ml of blood produces a fall in venous return, so reducing right ventricular output and causing a fall in mean capillary hydrostatic pressure.

Central venous or pulmonary artery catheterisation

These catheters may be inserted to aid the evaluation of the patient's haemodynamic status and to monitor the effects of medical interventions. Certainly inotropic drugs are best administered via a central route. However, it must be remembered that central venous pressure readings merely reflect activity on the right side of the heart and, as such, do not give any information on the functioning of the left side. Therefore, for this purpose, a pulmonary artery catheter may be used to provide indirect measurements of left atrial pressure and to show the pressure changes within the pulmonary circulation. However, specialised equipment and adequately trained staff to maintain them are required.

NURSING MANAGEMENT

Since the nurse is in constant contact with the patient and has the opportunity to observe him or her constantly, skilled observation can aid the rapid detection of early LVF. Observation and monitoring constitute the cornerstone of nursing in this situation.

Observation

The following signs and symptoms may indicate early heart failure.

Respiration

The onset of LVF is generally accompanied by a gradual increase in respiratory rate and degree of dyspnoea. Therefore it is important to observe respiratory status closely for signs of increasing respiratory rate. Also, the patient should be observed for increasing breathlessness, particularly with minimal exertion. The development of a cough, or worsening of a cough, may be an indication.

Heart rate

The development or persistence of a sinus tachycardia is suspicious of LVF, particularly if other causes can be excluded, e.g. pyrexia, anxiety or pain.

Sweating

Mild or moderate sweating, without any other obvious cause, may result from the increase in sympathetic stimulation that occurs when cardiac output falls.

Altered mentation

Although restlessness, anxiety and insomnia are common in hospitalised individuals, they may provide subtle clues to the development of LVF.

Treatment

During an acute episode of LVF and pulmonary oedema, the nursing aim is to ensure the smooth coordination of treatment and to support the patient and their family through this distressing episode, while monitoring the effectiveness of the medical treatment. Specific actions may be summarised as follows.

Positioning

Provided that the patient's ability to maintain their airway and consciousness level permits, they should be nursed in an upright position, preferably with their legs down. This not only improves ventilation by lowering the diaphragm but decreases venous return, so reducing preload.

Airway management

In severe cases, the airway may need to be maintained using an oropharyngeal or nasal airway, with the use of suctioning to clear secretions. It is sometimes necessary to secure the airway by endotracheal intubation and the use of positive-pressure ventilation to counteract the hypoxia.

Support

The inability to breathe properly stimulates a basic sense of fear and panic. This increases sympathetic stimulation further which exacerbates the condition. It may precipitate life-threatening dysrhythmias, caused by the sensitisation of the myocardium produced by the hypoxia. Any dysrhythmias that occur are treated according to the usual protocols. This demands a nurse skilled in providing psychological support, particularly if the patient is panicking or confused. Reassurance can be conveyed by the adoption of a calm, confident approach. Care should be planned to ensure that a nurse remains with the patient throughout the acute episode, not only for reassurance but to enable accurate and close monitoring.

Monitoring

Continuous cardiac monitoring should be established and maintained throughout the acute episode. This can be difficult to achieve because of the profuse sweating that accompanies acute pulmonary oedema, making electrode placement difficult. This permits the rapid identification of dysrhythmias, which occur frequently in the acute phase, from hypoxia or electrolyte imbalance. Basic evaluation of the patient's haemodynamic status may be made by observation of arterial blood pressure, heart rate and rhythm, urine output and skin temperature or skin feel. This is particularly important to ensure the patient's circulation is able to cope with the diuresis induced by the medical treatment. If central venous pressure or other more sophisticated techniques are being used, care must be planned in accordance with local protocols.

Generally, LVF responds well to treatment, provided that it is given in time, and provides the nurse with the satisfaction of seeing an acutely ill patient respond in a short space of time.

FURTHER READING

Canobbio M.M. (1990). *Cardiovascular Disorders*, Mosby, St. Louis.
Conway, N. (1977). *An Atlas of Cardiology*, Wolfe, London.
Meltzer, L. E., Pinneo, R., Kitchell, J. R. (1993). *Intensive Coronary Care: A Manual For Nurses*, Brady, Maryland.

Messineo F.C., Hage W.D. (1989). Haemodynamic complications of acute myocardial infarction. *Hospital Practice*, **24**(8): 147–162.

Thompson D.A. (1981).. *Cardiovascular Assessment: Guide for Nurses and Other Health Professionals*, Mosby, St. Louis.

White, B. S., Roberts, S. L. (1992). Pulmonary alveolar edema: preventing complications. *Dimensions Of Critical Care Nursing*, **11**(2): 90–103.

Wilson, D.D. (1989). Acute pulmonary oedema: how to respond to a crisis. *Nursing*, **19** (10): 34–42.

10.

FEAR OF DEATH

INTRODUCTION

Cardiovascular disease is so prevalent that few individuals will not have a family member, friend or colleague who has suffered from it and many will know of someone who has died from it. Ischaemic heart disease alone is responsible for over 160 000 deaths (roughly one every 3 minutes) and over 200 000 admissions to hospital annually in the UK. Fear of death is therefore a very real concern for cardiac patients and their families. It also poses a challenge for nurses (Thompson, 1994).

BACKGROUND

Death is the permanent cessation of all vital functions, the end of human life – an event and a state. Dying is a process of coming to an end, the final act of living. Fear is an unpleasant feeling caused by a threat in the environment that is specific and can be identified.

DEATH AND DYING

Although death is inevitable, the ways in which people view death and respond to the process of dying tend to be very individual. In the past, death was more common in infancy, childhood and young adulthood so people grew up surrounded by experiences of the death of peers, which forced them to reflect on their own mortality. Dying occurred frequently in the home and caring for the dying was a family experience. In modern Western society, characterised by an ageing population, death has tended to become institutionalised and far removed from normal experiences. In 1990 in England and Wales, one-quarter of deaths occurred in the person's own home, while nearly three-quarters occurred in institutions – most (54%) occurred in hospitals (OPCS, 1992). Faced with the possibility of death in themselves or others, individuals have very little to draw upon and no established networks of support. Feelings about death and dying therefore tend to be based upon ignorance and fear of the unknown. Such feelings will be influenced by factors such as age, experience and the perception of how real the threat or possibility of death is at that time.

Young adolescents may be unable to intellectualise their awareness of death and may isolate or repress their feelings about dying. Emotional awareness about their death is blocked by an inability to acknowledge the finality of their own existence. Young adults have developed ideas and concerns about death and dying. At this stage of human development, it is often not the actual death itself that causes concern but the process of dying. Feelings are related to pain, discomfort and fear of the unknown. Adults may not be so certain as they were in adolescence about whether there is life after death. The elderly often approach death in a calm manner, which is unusual in younger people. By this stage their enjoyment of life may have diminished and they are likely to have experienced the death of many family members and peers. An apparent acceptance of death may result from a desire to limit distress to family and friends and death may be preferred as an alternative to becoming useless and burdensome to one's family and society.

Attitudes to death are also influenced by current health status. Feelings to an abstract idea of an unknown death set at some as yet undetermined date far into the future are feelings towards an abstract death. Far more real are the feelings of those labelled with a medical diagnosis or condition who are forced to consider the implications of their new health status in terms of future lifestyle and possible mortality.

Most people viewing the subject of death from a detached distance state that they would prefer a sudden and unexpected death. However, the majority would also welcome the opportunity to say their 'goodbyes' to family and loved ones and to sort out their affairs beforehand. There is probably no such thing as an ideal death. The prospect of death and dying presents a unique challenge for individuals to draw on facets of their personality rarely tested and it is this challenge itself that evokes feelings of fear and foreboding for many.

DEATH AND THE CARDIAC PATIENT

The label 'cardiac patient' is an umbrella term covering a variety of medical conditions, each exerting a different impact upon the individual in terms of effect on lifestyle, perception of significance, outlook for the future and prognosis. The patient with angina is labelled with a diagnosis that may be transient or permanent. The impact of this diagnosis on the individual is likely to depend on a host of factors, including age of onset, severity of symptoms, degree of impairment, ability to cope, knowledge of the condition, experience of others with angina and the availability of support networks. Some individuals with angina choose to play down the significance of the condition and treat it as a minor inconvenience. Others make the condition the focus of their lives, controlling their thoughts and actions around avoiding symptoms, coping with symptoms and taking medication. Still others feel that they are only one step away from the inevitable heart attack that will kill them, so they place themselves in a long-term stressful situation where they are faced with the prospect of a sudden and unpredictable death. This has implications for long-term planning and roles within the family and workplace. It is also likely to affect the general mood and outlook of the individual and family.

The patient who has suffered a heart attack often views it as a 'bolt from the blue', particularly if previously fit and well, relatively young and consciously lead what he or she believes to be a healthy life. This can lead to feelings of anger, disbelief and denial. The patient with a history of angina may view his or her heart attack as something that was waiting to happen, nevertheless still experience feelings of shock and anger. Others with a history of angina perceive a heart attack as inevitable but probable relief of long-term symptoms. Indeed, some people with long-standing angina have an improved quality of life after suffering a heart attack. A heart attack is the leading cause of death in the UK and many people will know someone who has suffered or died as a result of one. In reality, most deaths from heart attacks occur in the first couple of hours after the onset of symptoms and it is not unrealistic to expect that most people who are admitted to hospital are likely to survive the event and resume a normal lifestyle. However, this does nothing to reduce the distress, particularly the anxiety and fear, that is present in the majority of patients and their loved ones on admission to hospital with chest pain. This anxiety may well still be significantly high on admission to the coronary care unit, on transfer from the unit to the ward, at the time of discharge and during early convalescence (Thompson, 1990). Sources of anxiety have been shown to revolve around personal relationships, return to work, activity and the future. Fear of death is probably behind many of these anxieties but it has not been addressed specifically as an issue in research literature, supposedly because of the sensitivity of the subject and the ethics of discussing the concept of death and dying with those striving for a successful recovery. Certainly, those patients and family members attending cardiac rehabilitation programmes frequently ask about the likelihood of a recurrence of a heart attack since there seems to be a prevailing notion that a first heart attack is a warning and that it is the second one that will kill them. This misconception must be a source of significant anxiety and fear for those who know that they have ischaemic heart disease. Such anxiety and fear may have a deleterious effect in terms of recovery. Fear of inducing a heart attack with its attendant risk of death is likely to incapacitate individuals in the normal fulfilment of many areas of their daily lives, such as work, leisure and sexual activity.

The small proportion of patients who have a heart attack and who then develop cardiogenic shock, who therefore have a poor outcome (a mortality rate of 90–100% within the first 24–48 hours), is perhaps the only group of cardiac patients where it is realistic to introduce the prospect of death at an early stage. These individuals and their loved ones are thus responding to fear of a death that is very real and immediate.

A further small proportion of cardiac patients who experience and survive a cardiac arrest are in a position where they often feel they have faced death and survived. Indeed, some such patients claim to have 'out of body experiences' characterised by leaving their body behind and travelling down a tunnel of light. Many patients claim to have been elevated above their hospital bed, a witness to their own resuscitation. Such experiences are bound to influence an individual's feelings about death and dying, often positively, with claims that the moment of death is no longer feared. Even cardiac arrest survivors who do not report such experiences (the majority) are likely to find themselves reflecting on the fact that they might have died and feel vulnerable, reconsidering their own feelings about death. Patients who witness a fellow patient suffer a cardiac arrest may worry that the same thing will happen to them. They may, however, feel reassured at the speed and competence of the resuscitation effort.

Cardiac patients requiring surgery, such as coronary artery bypass grafting, are in a position where they sense that something is being done to alleviate their symptoms. They are, however, faced with the concerns of other cardiac patients plus the added anxieties related to the surgical procedure and recovery process in a highly technical environment. Fears of receiving a general anaesthetic, of not waking up, of dying 'on the table' or in the immediate postoperative period, are likely to be experienced by many patients.

Patients with recurring, life-threatening, arrhythmias, particularly ventricular tachycardia, are often fearful of suddenly and unexpectedly losing consciousness as a result of a cardiac arrest. The level of fear is likely to depend on the individual's concept of the significance of the arrhythmia, past experience with treatment and confidence in current management regimes. Patients with implanted defibrillators, for example, suffer great psychological distress at being dependent upon a technical device. Likewise, patients fitted with cardiac pacemakers are faced with the prospect of death if there is an equipment malfunction.

FACTORS THAT INFLUENCE FEAR

Irrespective of the disease or disorder, the dying process is unique to each individual. Fear results from a person's familiarity and learned responses to previous negative experiences in life and observing the behaviour of others. Responses to death and dying are likely to depend on an individual's beliefs, attitudes and values. Death has real and symbolic significance in our society. It evokes questions about the meaning of life and poses ethical dilemmas about the quality of life, the 'right to know' and the duty to maintain life. Someone who believes that their life is preordained and who takes a fatalistic standpoint is likely to have different feelings from someone who feels they themselves have control over their own health problem and its outcome. Religious beliefs that provide solace in the concept of life after death or reincarnation may reduce fear in many, particularly if they believe that death will mean a reunion with their family and loved ones. Others may find their religious beliefs a source of anxiety as they ponder the prospect of judgement and having to answer for misdeeds performed in life. Secularisation of society has had an impact on our way of thinking about death. However, even those with no religious beliefs are likely to ponder the future and experience fear of the unknown.

Physical changes, both actual and anticipated, may evoke fear in some. The thought of changing body image, losing weight, nausea, vomiting, lethargy, altered mental state and, above all, pain and discomfort, and how they anticipate they will cope with them if and when the time comes, are important factors. The fear of losing control, regressing to a child-like state and being dependent upon others close to the time of death, may be a further cause of concern, as is loss of dignity, loss of identity and perceived decreased self-worth often associated with dying. Individuals may fear the actual moment of death as well as the process of dying and worry that they will be alone and fear abandonment and isolation.

Social and psychological support, actual and perceived, may both exacerbate and ameliorate the fear of death. Family members and loved ones are likely to experience similar fears to that of the patient. Strong family networks may offer support for offloading worries and concerns. Open lines of communication may help the individual feel that they are not facing the situation alone. Ideally, long-standing issues can be resolved and death can be faced with a feeling of completion and peace. Conversely, weaknesses in relationships and conflicts of roles may be magnified when the family unit is faced with the prospect of the death of a loved one and the family may become a source of stress. Attachment to others is a source of psychological strength and support but it is also a source of pain, loss and distress when there is a fear that these attachments are under threat. Individuals may fear the consequences of their death on those they are leaving behind. Concern about how a partner may manage emotionally, practically and financially, can add to the fear of dying itself. Anxiety about handing over responsibilities and roles to those whose competence is unknown or untested may result in further distress. Lack of trust in family members to carry out one's wishes compounds it.

Fears about death and dying are likely to change temporally as symptoms change, perceptions of illness are modified or as death itself draws closer. Awareness of the reality of impending death is also important. Glaser and Strauss (1965) identified four contexts in the awareness of dying:

- Closed awareness: the patient does not know he or she is dying but the staff (and possibly the family) know it. Fear of death is thus a reaction to a possibility at some unknown time.
- Suspected awareness: the patient does not know but suspects that he or she is dying. The staff and family know it. Pre-existing fears of death and dying are likely to be exacerbated by misconceptions and half-truths.
- Mutual pretence: the patient, staff and family know the patient is dying but there is tacit agreement to act as though this were not so. The patient may fear his or her approaching death but feel unable to express fear to others.
- Open awareness: the patient, staff and family know the patient is dying and act as if they do. Here, fear of death can be expressed if the patient feels able to do so.

The pattern of death will also influence an individual's feelings. Glaser and Strauss (1965) refer to the concept of dying trajectory and distinguish between 'quick' and 'slow' dying trajectories. Deaths that occur over a short space of time may well evoke greater fear than slow deaths, where patients have possibly been able to work through their fears.

MANIFESTATIONS OF FEAR

Fear of death and dying can manifest itself in a variety of ways affected by many factors including a person's developmental stage and ethnic and cultural background. Dying individuals experience several psychological reactions. Individuals who experience symptoms they fear may be serious, may deny their significance for fear of having to confront their own mortality. Many patients who have suffered a heart attack convince themselves that their pain is caused by indigestion or they try to ignore or work through the symptoms, hoping that they will go away. Delay in seeking medical aid and noncompliance with treatment are examples of behaviour of individuals who are afraid. Others who fear the consequences of their medical condition may seek medical help inappropriately, e.g. the patient with angina who telephones for an ambulance with every angina attack. Some demonstrate obsessive behaviour, where the potential life-threatening disorder becomes the focus of an individual's life, resulting in them thinking about medical treatment and prognosis at every opportunity. Being faced with the prospect of dying often leads to great sadness. There may be an urge to cry uncontrollably although there is frequently great pressure to be stoical and a fear of losing control. Feelings experienced may be frightening because of their intensity and unfamiliarity.

Kübler-Ross (1970) proposed that several stages could be identified in the psychological adjustment of patients once they knew they were dying:

- Denial and isolation: This stage is typically the initial reaction to the diagnosis of a terminal illness. It is the initial defence mechanism used to deal with news of impending death. It allows people to control the impact of bad news and come to an initial acknowledgement of it.
- Anger: This stage involves feelings of anger, rage and resentment as the dying person attempts to answer the question, 'Why me?' This anger can be directed at anyone and the more frightened the individual, the more angry he or she is likely to be.
- Bargaining: This stage includes an attempt to postpone the inevitable end much feared, by asking that the death be delayed in return for a particular promise. Bargains are often 'silent' or private.
- Depression: This stage begins when bargaining is seen as futile and is marked by two types of depression: reactive depression, resulting from issues that are experienced as part of the illness, and preparatory depression, which anticipates impending issues, such as separation from the family.
- Acceptance: This stage is marked by a degree of quiet expectation. Kübler-Ross stated that, provided patients have had enough time (i.e. not a sudden, unexpected death) and have been helped in working through their own response to dying, they will complete this stage.

Dying patients do not always progress through all these stages, nor in this order, and they may exhibit more than one reaction at a time. They often grieve in anticipation of the death itself and for the end of life. They may also withdraw from the surrounding social environment because of the fear of death and uncertainty as to how to react with others in their new role as someone who is dying. Hope, often present, even in those who realise the death they so fear is a great probability, is a powerful force that usually persists throughout the dying process.

MANAGING FEAR

If a patient recognises and acknowledges the specific cause of their fear it is possible for them or others to take action to reduce it. Fear of death and dying is likely to be reduced if the patient has a clear understanding of his or her health problem and its likely outcome and also a trust that they will be cared for in a manner that will minimise any distress.

Patients admitted to hospital with a suspected cardiac diagnosis such as a heart attack are likely to be reflecting on the seriousness of their condition and probably thinking that death is a very real threat. The highly technical environment of a critical care unit and the perceived serious condition of other patients is likely to exacerbate this threat. The hospital itself is associated with death for many who may recall visiting previously a terminally ill relative or witnessing the death of a fellow patient. Reducing a fear of death in this acute stage can be achieved by creating a calm, relaxed atmosphere for the patient and family where they feel valued, supported and able to be themselves and encouraged to ask questions and express their opinions (Thompson and Webster, 1992). Most patients admitted to hospital will not die and so stressing from the outset the fact that a good recovery is expected will aid in allaying fears. The death of a fellow patient can be particularly distressing, and reports of chest pain commonly increase after a cardiac arrest. This may make the patient and family wonder whether the same fate is likely to happen to the patient. Successful resuscitation of a fellow patient may prove reassuring for some patients but they are still likely to want an opportunity to discuss the matter. The subject of their own mortality may be discussed more easily in this sort of situation. Many patients who suffer a heart attack are young and have not previously been seriously ill. The sudden prospect of their own mortality being a potential reality is likely to be frightening and, not uncommonly, elicits feelings of hostility and denial. Time should be used carefully here as an opportunity for counselling and giving a realistic appraisal, clarifying issues and correcting misconceptions (Thompson, 1990).

Cardiac rehabilitation programmes provide an ideal opportunity in a controlled environment for offering such support and education. It is often during convalescence that fears and uncertainties manifest themselves, with individuals feeling vulnerable and worried about the rate at which they should resume activities and about the significance of their reactions and symptoms. Partners are often more worried than the patients (Thompson, 1990), feeling torn between appearing overprotective or not expressing enough concern. It is not uncommon for partners to engage in surveillance activities, secretly observing patients as they go about their daily activities. Night time is when most partners fear their loved one might die (in their sleep) and they often stay awake watching them. In order to bolster confidence and allay fear in cardiac patients and their partners, several simple measures can be taken (Thompson and Webster, 1992):

- Show a reassuring, concerned and positive attitude.
- Inform them of the cardiac disorder and its prognosis.
- Foster a realistic and optimistic outlook for the future.
- Stress to them that individuals vary in their response to cardiac disease.
- Prepare them for symptoms, such as chest pain, likely to be experienced and make them aware of their significance and management.
- Prepare them for mood changes, feelings of guilt, overprotectiveness, that are likely to be experienced.
- Offer them the opportunity to ask questions and discuss concerns.
- Provide them with honest and informed answers to specific questions.
- Involve family members so that they can be a source of support and prepare them for the possible effect of the cardiac condition on their relationships.
- Inform them of the importance of complying with treatments and attending follow-up appointments.

Cardiac patients tend to die either as a result of a cardiac arrest, or as a result of cardiogenic shock or heart failure, reflecting the fast and slow dying trajectories. A sudden death leaves little time for anticipation or fear but can leave relatives and health workers with a cocktail of emotions, including guilt, anger, helplessness, shock, denial and disbelief. A patient who is resuscitated successfully may fear a subsequent arrest with an unsuccessful outcome. Repeated resuscitation attempts may not be appropriate for some seriously ill patients and resuscitation that merely prolongs the process of dying would seem to be inappropriate in most cases. Deciding not to resuscitate is, of course, a controversial issue and the patient who becomes involved in this debate about their own life is faced with a complex range of arguments and counter-arguments that will be closely tied in with their attitudes about death and dying. Some patients will be unable to cope with such frank discussions about their own death and will need the support of a sensitive and highly experienced professional, such as a hospital chaplain, to act as a sounding board and advocate and, in some cases, to protect them from having to be involved in such decision-making.

Most patients become aware that they are dying even if the issue is not discussed with them. There is now a consensus that dying patients should be informed of their terminal condition for both moral and practical reasons. This is reflected in a move towards greater openness with the dying. It is argued that telling a patient they are dying allows open discussion, minimises mistrust and reduces patient loneliness and isolation and ultimately fear. Openness and honesty are important aids in assisting the terminally ill with their dying. However, when and how to disclose the bad news often remains a source of difficulty (Field, 1989).

The literature emphasises that effective communication influences the quality of the experience of dying and it may reduce fear. Both verbal and nonverbal communication are important in interactions with patients. Those caring for the dying should be able to recognise nonverbal signs of distress, a willingness to listen and information seeking, as well as to control their own signals to the patient. Patients tend to assume a passive role, do not want to appear to be a nuisance or to be ignorant, and hence are reluctant to ask questions or express concerns. Clear information devoid of ambiguity is essential to avoid the exacerbation of existing fears through misconceptions and hearsay.

To help a person die well is to support that person's sense of self-respect, dignity, control and choice until the final moment of life. Achieving this entails skilled and compassionate care designed to promote comfort and control suffering. Attending to physical needs, such as controlling pain and discomfort and promoting rest and sleep, are important ways of maintaining patient dignity, self-esteem and, if carried out, involve the patient in decision-making and a sense of control and purpose. High-quality care gives the patient the confidence that his or her needs will continue to be met when he or she is no longer in a position to taken an active involvement in his or her own care. Encouraging family members to be involved in physical care may reduce the fear they have of being with the dying person and give their visits purpose rather than sitting in awkward silence around the bed.

The dying patient is likely to require emotional support more than at any other time. Feelings of helplessness may cause them to depend on others to provide them with a sense of safety, security, love and warmth. Patients may find that they can only be themselves with a nurse or a relative stranger. The nurse can aid the patient and family by understanding common fears, facilitating communication and helping them accept reality. Patients may feel that their fears and concerns are trivial and unwarranted. Nurses can help patients by being open and uncritical, reassuring patients that such fears are common and by encouraging them to be expressed so that they can be dealt with.

Supporting the family is an indirect method of supporting the patient. Care designed to meet the needs of family members may enable the family to adapt and enhance their ability to support their critically ill relative. Family members are likely to have similar concerns and fears about death and dying and be fearful themselves both about the death of a loved one and the feelings evoked about their own death. Spouses in particular may experience intense feelings of loss from the perceived threat of their partner's death. Signs of fear and anxiety in the partner may evoke fears in the patient. Feeling involved and useful and being given a realistic appraisal of outlook are important. They should be given every opportunity to ask questions and express and discuss their worries and fears. Creating an environment where the patient and family feel welcomed, relaxed and uninhibited is important to reduce fear and to facilitate the expression of any fear experienced.

Patients who fear dying in the strange environment of a hospital and who express a wish to die at home should, where feasible, be given the resources and support to enable them to do so. This will involve close liaison with the family doctor, community nurse, social worker and other support agencies. Families need to be involved closely to ensure they can cope with having the patient home and so that problems can be anticipated and hopefully avoided.

To help a person die well is to support that person's sense of self-respecting dignity, control and choice until the final moment of life. Achieving this entails skilled and compassionate care designed to promote comfort and control suffering. Nurses are in an ideal position to get to know the patient and family and be there at times of need. They are also in a position to coordinate other support agencies such as that of spiritual support provided by the hospital chaplain.

Nurses may find it difficult to broach the subject of dying. They may use 'distancing tactics' to remove themselves from patients' and relatives' emotional suffering as a way of coping with the stress of the situation. Clearly, nurses must confront and reconcile their own fear of death and dying before they can help others effectively. Personal fear of death is related to anxiety about dealing with dying. An individual's experience of death, particularly the first experience of caring for a dying person, can be significant. Education, guided experience, peer support and a supportive work environment are ways of enabling nurses to cope. Nurses caring for cardiac patients are often geared to saving lives and may perceive death as a failure. Denial of the possibility of death means that strategies designed to minimise the fear of death in patients and families may not be in place. There may be difficulty in making the decision to move from treatment aimed at cure to palliative care aimed at symptom relief. Decisions to withhold resuscitation and to stop active treatment need to be discussed with all parties concerned, with the patient and family at the centre.

Field (1989) makes the important point that in critical care units, where many are managed, at least initially, cardiac patients are typically young and acutely ill, their stay short, 'recovery' and 'success' the norm and turnover rapid. The dying cardiac patient may be unconscious and be maintained on an aggressive treatment regime and, because the focus of nursing work is often highly specialised and of a medicotechnical nature rather than a psychosocial one, there is a danger that the dying patient is perceived as an anomaly.

REFERENCES

Field, D. (1989). *Nursing the Dying*, Tavistock/Routledge, London.

Glaser, B. G. and Strauss, A. L. (1965). *Awareness of Dying*, Aldine Press, Chicago.

Kübler-Ross, E. (1970). *On Death and Dying*, Tavistock, London.

OPCS (1992). *Mortality Statistics: General Review of the Registrar General on Deaths in England and Wales*. HMSO, London.

Thompson, D. R. (1990). *Counselling the Coronary Patient and Partner*, Scutari Press, London.

Thompson, D. R. (1994) Death and dying in critical care, in *Care of the Critically Ill Adult*, Millar, B. and Burnard, P. (Eds) Bailliere Tindall, London, pp. 234–249.

Thompson, D. R., Webster, R. A. (1992). *Caring for the Coronary Patient*, Butterworth-Heinemann, London.

11.

RESUSCITATION

It is now well accepted that the individual who falls victim to a cardiac arrest has the best chance of survival, not surprisingly, if being monitored in a high-dependency cardiac care area. However, the chances of survival from a life-threatening collapse can be improved if everyone in the now well-recognised chain of survival knows what to do. This chain includes the person who witnesses the collapse or is there very soon afterwards, the general practitioner, the ambulance service with defibrillators on board and the receiving emergency care area.

This chapter is aimed at refreshing basic knowledge, outlining the 1992 European Resuscitation Council Working Party recommendations (Chamberlain, 1992; Handley 1993, 1994) and identifying the need for regular resuscitation training for the multidisciplinary teams who may be dealing with people who could potentially collapse as a result of a cardiac arrest.

DEFINITIONS

There are a few definitions that might be considered:
- *Resuscitation* is 'the action of reviving from a state of apparent death' (*Odhams Concise English Dictionary*)
- *Cardiopulmonary resuscitation* can be defined as 'a technique employed to restore life or consciousness to a person apparently dead or dying, and includes external respiration and external cardiac massage' (Tortora, 1987).
- *Cardiac arrest* should be considered to be 'the cessation of mechanical cardiac activity as defined by loss of consciousness, absence of respiration and absence of a carotid pulse'.

INCIDENCE

When recognising the incidence of cardiac arrests several facts should be considered. There are thought to be over 160 000 deaths a year in the UK as a result of coronary artery disease; of these 50% die within the first 2 hours of the onset of symptoms. It is estimated that 70% of cardiac arrests occur in the home, thus the importance of teaching resuscitation skills to the public cannot be emphasised enough.

CAUSES OF CARDIAC ARREST

There are several reasons why a cardiac arrest may occur. The main precipitants are

- Airway obstruction.
- Hypoventilation.
- Electrocution.
- Poisons.
- Ischaemic heart disease.
- Sepsis.
- Hypovolaemia.
- Multisystem failure.
- Heart failure.

TO RESUSCITATE OR NOT

A major factor that must be taken into consideration in the hospital setting before subjecting the patient to what is a traumatic procedure for both the patient, the medical and nursing staff is whether or not the patient is actually considered to have any prospect of surviving an attempt of active resuscitation (Jones et al., 1993; Baskett, 1986,1993).

Points that should be taken into consideration when making such a decision of patients who are already in hospital are the patient's age, their past medical history. and their previous quality of life. This decision should be made under the guidance of the consultant in charge of the patient's care and members of the multidisciplinary team. Standing at the bedside of the patient is not the place to be making that decision. Similarly there is not enough time or space here to consider the full ethical implications of resuscitation but it is always something that should be considered and is currently under discussion by several authorities (Doyal *et al.*, 1993).

Factors to consider when patients are brought into hospital via the accident and emergency departments are the patient's age, any previous medical history if known. It is also important to try to establish how long the patient has been collapsed, if there was any bystander resuscitation and what treatment has been given by the paramedics at the scene (Skinner, 1991).

OUTCOME

A patient is more likely to survive a cardiac arrest if the event has been witnessed and resuscitation by a bystander commenced (Bossaert *et al.*, 1992; Tunstall-Pedoe *et al.*, 1992; Skinner and Vincent, 1993). The success of the arrest will be influenced by the cause of the collapse, which will have a better chance of success if the underlying reason for the collapse was ventricular fibrillation and if a defibrillator can be at hand to convert the electrical chaos of the myocardium to a sinus rhythm. There is a vast amount of work to support the role of early defibrillation.

Treatment of the individual who is a victim of a cardiac arrest falls into two parts: first, basic life support where no equipment is necessary a little skill and some basic knowledge is all that is required; second, advanced life support, which heralds the arrival of the ambulance service, paramedics or the cardiac arrest team, where there will be equipment and more knowledge and expertise.

RECOGNITION OF A CARDIAC ARREST

The diagnosis of a cardiac arrest must be made swiftly and accurately, i.e. the level of consciousness – whether conscious or not – and assessment of airway, breathing and circulation. To promote standard practice the European Resuscitation Council Working Party have produced a set of guidelines that should be followed by anyone teaching or performing resuscitation (Fig. 11–1). Probably the most important aspect of resuscitation is the prompt recognition of the condition accompanied by a call for help and activation of basic life support.

BASIC LIFE SUPPORT

This is easy to learn, and recall is considered easier and more effective if practised on a regular basis. On discovering the collapsed person, there should be prompt assessment using the standard ABC procedure.

Approach

A careful approach is needed. Is it safe for the patient and the rescuer? Consider hazards such as electricity, fumes and traffic.

Assess
Holding the victim by the shoulders shake gently and ask 'Are you alright?'. If there is no response, call for help.

Airway
This is one of the most important stages that must be performed efficiently and carefully. It should be performed by lifting the chin by placing two fingers on the chin which should pull the jaw forward then, by tilting the head with the other hand, the tongue should be lifted from the posterior pharyngeal wall. If any obvious obstruction is seen in the mouth, it should be removed. Care must be taken if there is any evidence to suggest a potential neck injury.

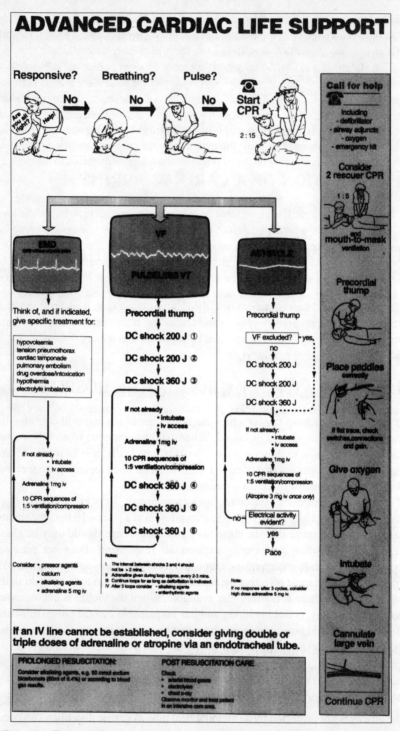

Fig. 11-1 European Resuscitation Council Working Party guidelines for resuscitation © ERC.

Breathing

Having cleared the airway, the victim's breathing must be assessed while keeping the airway open, this is performed by :

- Looking at the chest.
- Listening for any breath sounds.
- Feeling for any exhaled air.

This should take about 5 seconds. If the victim is breathing and it is clear that there are no spinal injuries, turn the person into the recovery position to prevent the airway from becoming obstructed and to allow any body fluids to drain away.

Circulation

Palpate the carotid pulse for 5 seconds.

DEALING WITH A PATIENT OUT OF THE HOSPITAL

Having performed the assessment described above, which should take no more than 15 seconds, the appropriate services should be called. If the subject is out of hospital an ambulance is required, which should be summoned as a matter of urgency.

DEALING WITH A PATIENT IN THE HOSPITAL

If the patient is in hospital, for which the remainder of the text will consider, the cardiac arrest team should be called. When sending someone to do this, ensure that they know how to do so and state the location clearly, it is of no use telling the switchboard operator that there is a 'cardiac arrest' then replacing the receiver. This is not the time or place for mystery and suspense!

When the victim is unconscious, has a clear airway, is not breathing but has a palpable carotid pulse, begin expired air respiration at a rate of 10 breaths/minute, taking care to observe that the chest rises and falls. There should only be slight resistance felt when performing expired air respiration. It is not pleasant performing mouth-to-mouth resuscitation and it only provides approximately 16% oxygen but is the most effective means of delivering oxygen to the victim in the situation where there is nothing else available. When the victim is unconscious, has a clear airway, is **not** breathing and has no palpable carotid pulse, full basic life support should be commenced, the ratios being as follows:

- Single rescuer: 2 breaths to 15 compressions.
- Two-person rescue: 1 breath to 5 compressions.

It can be hazardous to be over zealous in providing expired air respiration when the airway is not protected by an endotracheal tube as gastric distention can occur (Rimmer *et al.*, 1990), this in turn can cause gastric contents to be regurgitated and obviously increases the risk of aspiration.

The current anxieties regarding transmission of viral infections, particularly human immunodeficiency virus, to would-be rescuers is understandable but, to date, there has been no incidence of such an occurence. There is the facility to obtain very efficient airway adjuncts for such circumstances. This is discussed later in this chapter. Nevertheless, the health care worker who is exposed to the risk of being the first on the scene of a cardiac arrest more so than members of the public should be aware of the availability of equipment to be used as airway adjuncts within the hospital.

Chest compressions

Chest compressions should be performed by locating the correct position for the hands on the sternum. This is done by locating the xiphisternum, placing the middle finger at this point followed by the index finger, the heel of the other hand can then be placed above these landmarks and the first hand placed on top. The fingers of both hands are then interlocked to avoid pressure on the ribcage. The elbows are kept straight and the shoulders should be over the sternum to maximise the effort in depressing the sternum by 4–5 cm, which is repeated at a rate of 80 compressions/minute. There should be a pause between the breathing and compressions.

There are some developments in the delivery of chest compressions with the use of the Ambu Active compression decompression pump (Todd *et al.*, 1992). Thoughts behind such a device are to improve the intrathoracic pressure to improve the cardiac output and therefore produce a greater amount of blood transporting oxygen to brain cell. It is suggested that perfect chest compressions produce no more than 25% of normal cardiac output. Remember that the assessment of the patient, the recognition of the respiratory/cardiac arrest, calling for assistance and implementation of basic life support are essential if the patient is to stand any chance of survival.

The precordial thump in basic life support should only be considered if the collapse is witnessed or in a monitored situation. It is thought to be of little value in the unwitnessed collapse. It is suggested that there is up to a 25% chance of the thump converting apulseless ventricular tachycardia to sinus rhythm (Wynne, 1993).

It is essential that all nurses are trained in resuscitation skills on a regular basis as research has shown that these skills deteriorate if not practised (David and Prior-Willeard, 1993; Berden *et al.*, 1993). The opportunity to practice resuscitation skills has been improved considerably over the past few years with the development of the role of the resuscitation training officer, and rooms dedicated for resuscitation training plus an ever-increasing range of sophisticated training equipment. There are, however, several problems to overcome in ensuring that everyone is not only trained but updated on a regular basis. There are areas in other countries where, to practise as a doctor or nurse, an annual cardiopulmonary resuscitation assesment assessment has to be taken. If this were the case in the UK, many more resuscitation training officers would have to be appointed but it would certainly help raise standards, and indeed levels of awareness, in this crucial area.

BASIC LIFE SUPPORT IN THE HOSPITAL

It is the nurse's responsibility to know for which patients active cardiopulmonary resuscitation would be an inappropriate course of treatment. The area in which the patient may collapse should be made as suitable as possible for resuscitation to be performed. If the bed is too high and cannot be lowered, suitable stools or steps should be made available to stand on. Care is needed when considering the possibility of a patient on a specialised low air flow or air-cushion bed, although these generally have cardiopulmonary resuscitation functions to allow the bed to be made firm or to be deflated. These are adequate functions but have the potential to be quite alarming if not practised before the event. Actions such as removing the back off the bed and removing furniture that could be in the way are important points for all members of staff. In addition, all members of staff must know the hospital cardiac arrest number and from where to collect the emergency equipment.

Airway adjuncts

Barrier devices

The first to consider is the barrier devices, such as the Laerdal face shield (Fig. 11-2), or the Ambu Life Key (Fig. 11-3). Both provide a layer of plastic between

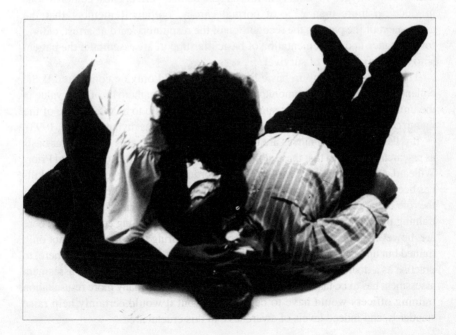

Fig. 11-2 Use of a barrier device - the Laerdal face shield © Laerdal Medical.

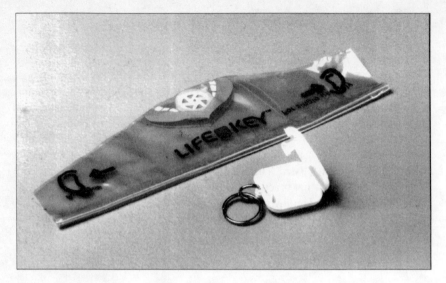

Fig. 11–3 The Ambu Life Key © Ambu International UK.

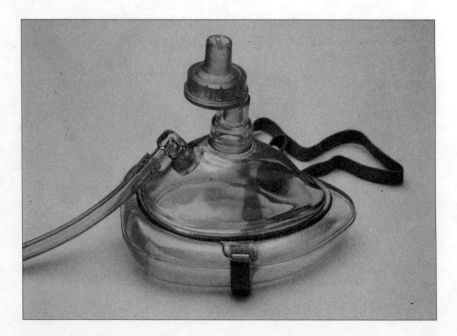

Fig. 11–4 The Laerdal pocket mask © Laerdal Medical.

the rescuer and the victim and filter the rescuer's breath and divert any body fluids from the victim away from the rescuer. With both of these, the filter should be placed over the victim's mouth. There will possibly be air that escapes from around the edge but both are excellent pieces of first-aid equipment when being confronted unexpectedly by a collapsed apnoeic individual, particularly because they are small and compact and therefore easy to carry around.

Mask devices

The leading mask device is the Laerdal pocket mask (Fig. 11-4). This is packaged in a collapsed state in a small container and is ideal to be carried in the pocket of a white coat, briefcase or in the car. It is moulded in such a way that it will fit any face size when placed correctly. This allows for good management of the airway by providing a jaw lift and application of expired air respiration via the mouthpiece with or without the optional filter, so avoiding direct mouth-to-mouth contact. There is also a more sophisticated device available that has a head strap and an inlet for oxygen to enrich the exhaled air from the rescuer.

While being a very handy first-aid device they really should be sited close to patient areas if not above every patient's bed, rather than on the arrest trolley, which is equipped with far more equipment.

Guedal airway

This should be inserted into the mouth of the unconscious person to assist in maintaining a clear airway by reducing the occlusion of the airway by the unconscious floppy tongue. The size should be assessed carefully as a short guedal airway only serves to further obstruct the airway by pushing the tongue back even further. If the airway is too long it will occlude the airway by pushing the epiglottis back.

Bag–valve–mask device

In hospital situations, the most commonly used piece of equipment should be the bag–valve–mask device. This device allows, at worst, room air to be squeezed into the victim's lungs, with the option of improving oxygenation by adding oxygen. Its use is improved by delegating one person to hold the mask, using both hands to provide a jaw thrust and a seal with the mask on the patient's face, while a second person squeezes the bag to inflate the chest. This is not a technique to be attempted by inexperienced staff. The effectiveness is increased further when there is a Guedel airway *in situ*.

Advanced cardiac life support

This is distinguished by the arrival of the cardiac arrest team supported by the emergency equipment namely oxygen, suction, defibrillator and drugs.

Equipment

Too much equipment is not only bulky and confusing but it is potentially expensive. The equipment for each area should, wherever possible, be standardised within the hospital to avoid confusion among staff moving to different areas. The

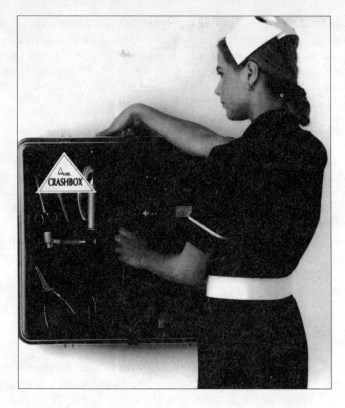

Fig 11–5 Storage of equipment together in a secure yet accessible place is essential © Rhesus Positive Ltd.

basis for the selection of equipment should be that there is enough to cover the range of potential emergencies without having three or four of the same items 'just in case'. The equipment should be stored together securely, yet be accessible where everyone working within that area knows where to obtain it (Fig. 11-5).

ADVANCED CARDIAC LIFE SUPPORT

The European Resuscitation Council Working Party put together the Advanced Resuscitation Guidelines. The function of the guidelines is to provide simple, easy-to-follow algorithms for each of the three most likely cardiac rhythms present at a cardiac arrest. The cardiac arrest should be managed in a confident, clear and calm manner. The organisation of the team at the event is the task of the team leader.

Team approach to the management of a patient in cardiac arrest

For each patient who has a cardiac arrest the aim is to restore a cardiac output as soon as possible so that there is no neurological deficit. In order to achieve this, the procedure should be a well-rehearsed and practised performance. It is understandable that staff working in areas where the are few cardiac arrests are anxious about the event; however, with regular training the scenario is less daunting and should help reduce anxiety.

It is important that someone arrives to take control and conduct the crisis in an organised fashion. Sadly this is often not the case; however, with resuscitation training having a higher profile and with the publication of guidelines this should eventually happen.

The resuscitation team should have designated tasks, these can be distinguished broadly as follows:

- *Team leader*: Coordinates activity and gathers information regarding the patient's medical history, current illness, makes decisions and controls the 'crowd' at the bedside. It is the team leader's responsibility to ensure that the team members are coping with their role and, if necessary, offers a substitute for tiring tasks such as providing external chest compressions.
- *Doctor 1*: Intubates and creates a central venous access.
- *Doctor 2*: Defibrillates and creates a peripheral venous access.
- *Nurse 1*: Gives external chest compression.
- *Nurse 2:* Attaches monitor, clears bed area and collects other equipment as required.
- *Nurse 3*: Prepares drugs and records events, should probably be the most senior nurse at the scene.

THE MOST COMMON RHYTHMS CAUSING CARDIAC ARREST

These are ventricular fibrillation, asystole and electromechanical dissociation. They are all life-threatening, having no palpable cardiac output.

Ventricular fibrillation

The most common and certainly the most treatable is ventricular fibrillation, it may present initially as pulseless ventricular tachycardia, often without a palpable pulse. When a cardiac arrest is identified, the priority is to defibrillate as soon as possible. Pulseless VT, usually with a rate greater than 180 beats/minute demands the same urgency as ventricular fibrillation because of the nature of the loss of cardiac output from which the patient will lose consciousness rapidly. The baseline observation to use with any emergency is the state of the patient. It must be stressed that the patient should be checked as well as the monitor.

The importance of early defibrillation must be emphasised and the sequence of three prompt shocks at 200, 200 and 360 Joules should be second nature followed by the recurring loop of intravenous adrenaline (1 mg)* and then three further shocks at 360 Joules should be repeated for as long as is necessary.

Asystole

Since this lack of electrical activity has such a poor prognosis, care should be taken to establish that it really is a straight line rather than fine ventricular fibrillation, which if defibrillated carries a higher chance of reverting to a rhythm with an output.

Having confirmed that it is asystole, the priority should be to provide oxygenation by intubation. Venous access should be established and 1 mg of adrenaline administered.* Following at least 10 cycles of basic life support, the one dose of atropine (3 mg) should be given. If there is any response and a palpable carotid pulse produced, it might be necessary to consider pacing. In the absence of success, further doses of adrenaline should be given.

Electromechanical dissociation

Here the electrical activity of the heart continues but with no palpable pulse. This may be the result of failure of the myocardium or a secondary reason such as hypovolaemia, drug overdose, tension pneumothorax, cardiac tamponade or hypothermia. In these situations the primary treatment must be to treat the cause. The drug treatment of electromechanical dissociation should be as before, 1 mg of adrenaline in this case for cardiac support, if treating the cause is successful.

This is the only rhythm for which calcium is considered and then only as a result of the cause being suspected as an overdose of calcium-channel-blocking drugs, or for hyperkalaemia or hypocalcaemia.

DEFIBRILLATION

As a result of the many studies that have demonstrated the importance of early defibrillation, it is vital that the patient is offered the best chance of survival by having the equipment and personnel to provide this service. It is clear that since nurses are often first to discover the patient and administer basic life support they should be the individuals to defibrillate the patient, since it is the treatment that should be administered with minimum delay. This is seen in many areas as an extended role for the nurse and suitable training is provided, sadly in others it is not seen as a nursing task.

There are several types of defibrillators on the market, basically manual and advisory. The latter do the thinking and advise that a shock is suitable for the

---

*The dose of adrenaline may be doubled or trebled and administered down the endotracheal tube in the event of an intravenous line being difficult to insert.

detected rhythm. Whichever device is used, there are several considerations that should be made before defibrillating the patient, namely:

- Check the patient is in ventricular fibrillation and hence needs to be defibrillated.
- Remove patient's clothing from the chest.
- Apply gel pads or gel to prevent burns to the skin.
- Check for pacemakers, in particular the generator type.
- Check the chest for GTN patches and remove (the aluminised patches can explode).
- Dry the patient's chest if moist and ensure that the operator is not standing in water.
- Avoid placing paddles over the ECG electrodes.
- Before delivering the shock tell everyone to 'stand clear'.

Paddle placement

The position of the paddles on the victim's chest is important since it influences the current flow through the myocardium. To be effective with the delivery of the shock, a critical mass of fibrillating heart muscle needs to be depolarised so that conduction can take over from the sinoatrial node. To maximise the effect of the shock, one paddle should be placed below the outer half of the right clavicle and the other at the area of the V4 and V5 chest lead positions and firm pressure applied to each paddle as the discharge buttons are pressed.

Despite clear labels on the paddles of many defibrillators, it is misleading since it is not vital which is placed in the apex or sternal region; additionally the paddle should not be placed over the sternum since the bone offers appreciable resistance to the current. If, however, when the paddles are being used to monitor the patient they are placed in the wrong position, the complex will be seen to be upside down.

Endotracheal intubation

This is the optimum means of managing the airway of the unconscious patient in the event of a cardiac arrest. However, it is a specialised skill that is difficult for the untrained person to perform, and therefore should not be attempted by anyone who has not successfully intubated before. Indeed, if the endotracheal tube cannot be inserted in less than 30 seconds it should be abandoned and the patient oxygenated by one of the other methods.

Intravenous access

It should be standard practice at the cardiac arrest that all first-time drugs are injected into either a peripheral line, preferably the antecubital fossa, or into a central venous line.The internal jugular and subclavian veins are the central lines recommended for emergency cannulation. There are, however, more potential complications using a central venous route. Among these are haemorrhage, pneumothorax or sepsis. A small cannula in the back of the patient's hand is not an acceptable route at this time since the drug will be unlikely to enter the central circulation and hence be of little benefit to the patient.

Improving survival figures

Many more lives could be saved if there were more individuals who were able to administer basic life support. This figure could be also be improved if individuals were more aware of recognising the symptoms and significance of chest pain and therefore sought advice appropriately (Baskett, 1992; David and Prior-Willeard, 1993; Berden et al., 1993).

With the development of more advance life-support courses under the direction of the Resuscitation Council (UK) there should be an improvement in the standard of resuscitation training, which has been questioned in some areas (Kaye et al. 1991; Wynne et al., 1992; Smith, 1993) and therefore improve the delivery of immediate care to victims of cardiac arrest. The importance of regular repeated resuscitation training for all individuals cannot be emphasised enough, more so for all staff working with patients who are likely to collapse, since it is too easy to learn bad habits by following a poor role model. The survival figure highlights the point that resuscitation has a long way to go before we get it right.

Caring for the carers

In the period after the arrest there will be activity; either stabilising the patient and arranging transfer to high-care areas or, if rescussitation was unsuccessful, dealing with relatives and tidying up the bed area. It is all too common that there is no time taken to talk through the events with those involved at the time, e.g. the nurses and doctors. This is an ideal time for team debriefing to air thoughts and feelings that, if dealt with at the time, can reduce the stress and anxiety produced by these situations and assist in improving standards of care and skill.

REFERENCES

Baskett, P.J.F. (1986). The ethics of cardiopulmonary resuscitation.British Medical Journal, **293**: 189–190.

Baskett, P.J.F. (1992). Teaching the public CPR. British Journal of Hospital Medicine **48** (8): 447–451.

Baskett, P. J. F.(1993). Ethics in cardiopulmonary resuscitation. Resuscitation, **25**: 1–8.

Berden, H., Williems, F., Hendrick, J., et al. (1993). How frequently should basic cardiopulmonary resuscitation training be repeated to maintain adequate skills? British Medical Journal, **306**: 1576–1577.

Bossaert, L., Koster, R. (1992). Defibrillation: methods and strategies. Resuscitation, **24**: 211–225.

Chamberlain, D.(1993). for the European Resuscitation Council, Adult advanced life support: the European Resuscitation Council Guidelines 1992 (abridged). *British Medical Journal*, **306**: 1589–1593.

David, J. and Prior-Willeard, P. (1993). Resuscitation skills of MRCP candidates. *British Medical Journal*, **306**: 1587–1579.

Doyal, L. and Wilsher, D. (1993). Withholding cardiopulmonary resuscitation: proposals for formal guidelines. *British Medical Journal*, **306**: 1593–1596.

Handley, A.(1993). for the European Resuscitation Council, Basic Life Support Working Group. Guidelines for Basic Life Support *British Medical Journal*, **306**: 1587–1589.

Handley, J. (1994) Guidelines for advanced life support. European Resuscitation Council Guidelines. *Resuscitation, ***23**(2): 111–122.

Jones, A., Peckett, W., Clark, E., *et al.* (1993). Nurses' knowledge of the resuscitation status of the patients and action in the event of cardiopulmonary arrest. *British Medical Journal*, **306**: 1577–1578.

Kaye, W., Rallis, S. F., Mancini, M. E. *et al.* (1991). The problem of retention of Cardiopulmonary resuscitation skills may lie with the instructor, not with the learner or the curriculum. *Resuscitation*, **21**: 67–87.

Rimmer, J. A. P., Smedley F. H., Allen-Marsh, T. G. (1990). Gastric Rupture following cardiopulmonary resuscitation. *ITMC*, **Nov-Dec**: 210–213.

Skinner, D. V. (1991). Management of cardiac arrest. *Hospital Update*, **5**: 415–419.

Skinner, D.V., Vincent, R. (1993). *Cardiopulmonary Resuscitation*. Oxford University Press.

Smith C. (Editorial) (1993). Better resuscitation training needed. *British Journal of Nursing*, **2**(1): 5.

Todd, J., Cohen, M. D. (1992). Active compression-decompression. A new method of cardiopulmonary resuscitation. *Journal of the American Medical Association*, **June**: 3.

Tortora, Anagnastakos; *Principles of Anatomy and Physiology*. Fifth Edition. Harper and Row Publishers, New York

Tunstall-Pedoe, H., Bailey L., Chamberlain, D. A., *et al.* (1992). Survey of 3765 Cardiopulmonary resuscitations in British Hospitals (the BRESUS study): methods and overall results. *British Medical Journal* **304**: 1347–1351.

Wynne, G. (1993). Revival techniques.*Nursing Times*, **89** (11): 26–31.

Wynne, G., Marteau, T. and Evans, T. R. (1992). Instructors – a weak link in resuscitation training. *Journal of Royal College of Physicians*, **26**: 372–373.

ONGOING PATIENT CARE

12.

PATIENT EDUCATION

Recent government initiatives have raised the priority for the need for patient education. The *Patient's Charter* (Department of Health, 1991) emphasises the patient's right to be informed about treatments patients may receive. The *Health of the Nation* (Department of Health, 1992) set targets for the improvement of health related to specific conditions in the population of the UK. For coronary artery disease, there is a stated aim to reduce the number of deaths of people under 65 years by 40% by the year 2000. The nurse's role has been stated clearly in the *Strategy for Nursing* (Department of Health, 1989):

'health education and promotion should be a recognised part of health care; all practitioners should develop skills in and use every opportunity for health promotion'.

Therefore nursing has a prime role in the education of patients. This is logical as the nurse is the carer with the most contact with the patient and highest profile.

NURSING ASSESSMENT

A myocardial infarction is a life-threatening condition with major implications for the patient's return to a full and active life. Therefore, providing the patient and his or her family with information, guidance and support from the early admission phase through to full recuperation is essential. However, the nurse faces difficulties in meeting these needs. Following a myocardial infarction the patient is placed suddenly into a threatening environment where the prospect of death is very real. Wilson-Barnett (1984) identifies three elements of stress that can affect patients following hospitalisation:

- Threat of the unknown, i.e. pain, severity of illness.
- Loss of health, independence, liberty and company.
- The challenge to behave well and be a good patient.

These elements will be apparent to a greater or lesser degree at different stages during the patient's hospital stay. Each will give rise to varying levels of anxiety, which will hinder the patient's ability to absorb information. The nurse must be aware of the stresses placed upon the patient when planning any educational input. An example of this is the resentful patient who is constantly asking 'Why me?' following his or her infarct. Jacobsen *et al.* (1992) reported high levels of anxiety in patients such as this in the early phase of admission following a myocardial infarction. This is where patient education, being mistakenly seen as shorthand for 'risk factor modification', can be most apparent. The nursing assessment of the patient's educational needs must include the necessity of helping him or her to cope with the anger and injustice that he or she feels.

The general reduction in the length of hospital stays will also present the nurse with a problem in meeting the patient's needs. Many nurses will identify with the situation where patient education is one action among many. Lipetz *et al.* (1990) found that nurses spent 8% of their time on patient education. It is likely, however, that the patient teaching was in formal, planned sessions, ignoring the high level of informal contact during which much information is passed.

The situation of patient teaching competing with other nursing responsibilities has led, in part, to the creation of specialist nursing posts particularly in diabetic and cardiac nursing. The role played by the clinical nurse specialist in patient education is vital but can only be fully effective if this nurse works closely with the rest of the care team.

The time factor will influence the nursing assessment of what is realistic and necessary for the patient to learn during his or her stay in the hospital. This must be, as Daniels *et al.* (1988) points out, a two-way dialogue. The temptation here is for nurses to teach patient what they feels patients ought to know. This is obviously to be avoided since the nurse's perception of what subjects are important are likely to differ to that of the patient. For example, Chan (1990) found that patients rated very low the importance of learning what the heart looks like and how it works. This may be surprising since nurse training was often based on learning the normal before understanding the abnormal. Further difference in perception between nurses and patient can be in the level of understanding of information given. Wallace *et al.* (1985) investigated this issue in a coronary care setting and found that, while nurses performed well in assessing the patient's information needs, they were less accurate in assessing the patient's understanding of the information The process of assessment must be ongoing and repetition and further explanation will be necessary. It is perhaps best to work on the assumption that the patient will absorb approximately 30% of the information given to him or her.

Any educational input will be depend greatly on the patient's willingness to learn about his or her illness and recovery. The nursing plan should not be based on the patient's obligation to learn. Lipetz *et al.* (1990) see this obligation as a method of blaming the patient for the illness. The burden of guilt that may ensue may be difficult for the patient to cope with as well as other emotions he or she may be experiencing, such as fear, confusion and anger. This may lead to a period of denial, which will need to be overcome before any educational input can be effective.

The debate on the beneficial or negative effects of denial on the patient's recovery remains inconclusive (Lowery, 1991, 1992; Malan, 1992; Russell, 1993). Whether it acts, for example, as a buffer to the reality of the situation or leads to poor patient compliance in the long term is unclear. As carers, it leaves us on uncertain ground as to how to deal with the situation. While patients will have difficulty sustaining denial of the fact they have had a heart attack because of the constant remainders surrounding them in the coronary care unit (Johnson and Morse, 1990), many will frequently experience some denial of the effect of their heart attack. This is a situation in which a degree of collusion between the patients and carers often occurs; witness the number of patients who will say they have been told they have had a 'small heart attack'. This collusion can be defended to a point as a means of sustaining vital hope in the patient. However, the need to adopt a positive approach with the patient, highlighting what he or she can do rather than the limitations, must be tempered by a degree of realism.

After identifying the patient's need for education, it is essential to consider the needs of the patient's partner and family. While the initial needs will be similar to those of the patient, there will quickly be longer-term concerns, summarised by Nyamathi (1990), i.e. personality changes in the patient, role changes in the family, financial insecurity, resumption of sexual activity, vagueness in the physician's instructions, lack of knowledge and information about their relative's condition, the possibility of a recurrent event and dealing with an uncooperative partner. A separate nursing plan may be needed to meet the family's needs.

THE NURSING PLAN

The goals of a nursing plan will be to help patients and their families understand the nature of the disease, to help them to understand the treatments and investigations they may undergo and to help them achieve the lifestyle adjustments that may be necessary. A nursing plan must take into account the patient's changing needs as he or she progresses through the hospital stay. It must also address the individual needs of the patient. Certain information will be more relevant at different stages during the patient's recovery.

One suggested framework in which patient teaching can be given in this staged manner is to divide the patient's recovery up into three phases. This method is described by Moynihan (1984, citing original work by Comoss 1979).This is the structure that will be used in this chapter when discussing nursing intervention..

Phase 1 of patient teaching begins with the patient's admission to the coronary care unit and continues until the patient's transfer to the general medical ward or cardiac ward. It is here that phase 2 begins; it continues until the patient is discharged home. Phase 3 begins after the patient's discharge and continues until he or she has returned to a normal lifestyle. The content of the plan will depend on the patient's general needs, the identified individual needs and the resources available to the nurse.

Nursing intervention

Phase 1

Previous reference to the levels of stress the patient will be placed under just by being admitted to hospital, has been made. With particular reference to phase 1 of the patient education plan, mention must also be made of the prehospital experience common to many patients. The patient arriving on a coronary care unit is likely to have experienced a sudden episode of severe chest pain, which heralds the start of a threatening experience over which he or she has little control. The patient is rushed to hospital in an ambulance, received into a specialised room surrounded by unfamiliar 'high-tech' equipment and transferred to a special unit to be cared for by specialist staff.

While all these actions are fully justified and necessary for the patient's medical care from the point of view of patient teaching, it often leaves us with the starting point of a patient who has had the severity of his or her condition demonstrated graphically. The patient is suddenly aware of his or her finite existence and has surrendered independence and control of his or her life to carers in whom he or she now places an enormous amount of trust.

Patient teaching in this phase begins as soon as the patient is ready. The initial need is to build up a rapport with the patient and family. Despite efforts to reduce the threatening appearance of coronary care and intensive care units, these environments can still appear alien to many people. Therefore brief and simple explanations of equipment around the patient's bed, with their unfamiliar noises and flashing lights, is essential. To the patient's family, the cardiac monitor is often a source of great comfort and, conversely, anxiety. It provides them with physical confirmation that their loved one's heart is still beating. Subsequent disturbance of the tracing by the patient moving can be a source of great worry and requires gently encouragement from the nurse for them to look at the patient rather than the equipment.

When the patient's condition stabilises to the point where he or she is free of pain and is no longer under the influence of narcotic analgesia, the trust and rapport that has been built up will be of positive benefit as the patient's education becomes more formalised. The patient will often want to make some sense of the situation which he or she now finds himself (herself) in and a good starting point can be to allow the patient to speak fully about the events leading up to his or her admission, the feelings of pain, fear and impending death. This can provide the nurse with valuable clues about the patient's response to their heart attack, e.g. the degree of denial, if any, felt by the patient, the patient's thoughts on possible causes of his or her heat attack, the reaction and needs of their close family and other emotions they may be feeling such as guilt or anger.

For some patients, the most relevant issue at this stage is that of survival, the need is to know what has happened, what treatment is required and what actions can they take to prevent it happening again. For others, the fear of death may not be so apparent (Shearck, 1992) because of confidence in modern technology and the abilities of the staff caring for them. Retention of information from the previously discussion on anxiety is often very low so repetition of information is essential. A simple description of what happened to the heart during a heart attack can be given by using a picture or diagram showing the heart muscle and coronary arteries. The use of a model heart may be considered, although patients often feel quite threatened by these. The need is for the patient to understand what has happened. This will provide him or her with a basis to relate other advice and information given. A description of the drug therapies, investigations and likely length of stay in hospital can also be discussed at this stage. If relevant, emphasis may be placed on a description of the use of thrombolitic therapy, as the patient may see this as a positive intervention to reduce the severity of the heart attack.

By this stage, the patient may have started to ask the question 'Why?' and to consider what action to take to prevent a recurrence. If the patient has decided on healthier options, the nurse can confirm the benefits of these changes and discuss what care may be available to help the patient achieve these objectives in the longer term. The nurse may also act as a guide if appropriate for the patient to identify or modify a risk factor in his or her lifestyle, e.g. smoking. The nurse must also consider the patient who does not have an easily identifiable risk factor present in his or her lifestyle. This patient is not presented with the option of having something to do about his or her predicament, the need is then to help the patient deal with the feelings of anger and resentment felt.

Phase 2

The move from the coronary care unit to the general ward can be a fraught time for the patient and his or her family. The initially threatening environment of the coronary care unit has become one of great security. Anxiety levels are likely to be raised and the patient will need time to settle into the new environment before he or she feels ready to take in any further information. As the acute phase of the patient's illness recedes, consideration of issues related to the longer-term recovery become more relevant. It is likely that the family will have reached this phase earlier than the patient as they make plans for the future. This is where the importance of the assessment phase is apparent so that the individual's needs are met at the appropriate time.

Specific advice is needed on any lifestyle adjustments that may be necessary. To help the patient reduce a risk factor in his or her lifestyle, the nurse must take the wider view of the patient's life and consider reasons for the patient indulging in a particular behaviour. In the case of smoking, the nurse can emphasise the importance of giving up smoking and discuss the patient's feelings about this. The patient will also need further guidance on ways of stopping smoking and what support services may be available following discharge. There may be reasons behind the patient's smoking and these will need to be discussed. If there is a strong social factor, referral to a social worker and liaison with patient's general practitioner will be appropriate. While any change in the patient's lifestyle depends on motivation to change, the nurse can do more than advise. With the patient's need for specific advice at this phase in his or her care, it is helpful to use other specialist services such as a dietician.

Other subjects related to the return to normal life are general activity and exercise, emotional response, family relationships and resumption of sexual activity, returning to work, driving and advice on holidays and flying. The patient and his or her family will probable be unsure about resuming some of these activities, in particular returning to work. Patients may make an early decision that they may need to change their job or perhaps will never be able to work again. In the long term, for a minority of patients, this may turn out to be true but early decisions like this are often made on the assumption that, after a heart attack, they will never be the same again. Along with reinforcing the message that a return to normal life is possible, the patient needs help to understand that being in hospital places him or her in a very false environment and major changes like this, which are difficult enough, need to be made when the patient and family have had time for discussion and readjustment back into their home environment.

The response when advising patients about the return to their sex life may vary at this stage. Some patients may not feel this is relevant. This can give the nurse the wrong impression that patients do not view this subject as particularly relevant or important. It is essential, therefore, that this subject is included in phase 3 of the educational plan and included in the written material supplied.

As the discharge date draws near, specific guidance is needed for the early period following discharge. The family are taking on the role of the principle carer, which they may feel poorly prepared for, and will need information regarding medications, what to do in the event of further symptoms, what role the GP plays in the patient's care and who to contact should they have any questions. Discharge from hospital is a worrying time for the patient and the family. The value of good communication between them should be stressed to try to avoid the conflicts and frustrations that may arise if the patient feels over protected. Information about the cardiac rehabilitation service should be given along with an agreed date for the patient's first attendance. It may also be helpful to arrange to phone the patient and his family on an agreed date, say one week after discharge, just to discuss their progress. A visit to the patient's home may be negotiated if resources allow.

Phase 3

Patients will attend the cardiac rehabilitation course usually a week or two following discharge. Cardiac rehabilitation is discussed in the next chapter. As part of phase 3 of the patient educational programme, it will probably be the first time that the patient is involved in group discussion. There will also be the added influence of the patient's and family's experiences following discharge. Up until this stage, they may have thought the problems and worries that they have had have been individual to them and being in a group environment will often help them to realise the similarity of their experiences to others and a degree of peer support can be given.

The content of the educational programme at this stage will be similar to that discussed in the previous two phases; however, as the patient is now in a much less stressful situation, the value of teaching in the outpatient phase is much higher (Marshall *et al.*, 1986; Steele and Ruzicki, 1987). Again the balance must be on risk factor modification and resuming normal life activities. Suggested content of a twice weekly 6-week programme is:

- The heart, its structure, function, what happens in a heart attack.
- Emotional reaction to heart problems.
- Diet, different food groups, what are fats?
- Diet, changing to healthy eating.
- Role changes.
- Exercise and the heart.
- Stress, what is it, how does it affect us?
- Stress, suggested coping strategies.
- Resuming sexual activity.
- Medications and the heart.
- Educational video followed by discussion.
- Evaluation.

The value of group discussion within this framework cannot be over-emphasised. The programme is also supplemented by less formal discussion with the patient and family about any individual concerns they may have. Phase 3 will end according to the patient's needs. In some cases it will finish at the completion of the cardiac rehabilitation programme, in others who are requiring long-term help to change a risk factor within their lifestyle, e.g. smoking, which may continue until that objective is achieved.

EVALUATION OF CARE

The majority of the nursing goals are long term, therefore true evaluation of the nursing intervention will involve contacting the patient again after a set period of time to assess the extent to which patients have adapted their lives and, if appropriate, modified risk factors within their lifestyles. While the effect on patient compliance is variable (Marshall *et al., 1986*; Penckofer and Llewellyn, 1989; Miller *et al.*, 1990), the degree to which the patient has regained control of his or her life is highly relevant (Johnson and Morse, 1990). Short-term evaluation can be carried out when assessing the patient's level of knowledge and achieving specific goals of returning to normal lifestyle activities, e.g. driving and, where appropriate, returning to work. Subjective evaluation of the patient's and family's feelings of well-being and ability to cope with differing demands placed upon them, especially in the early discharge days, is also relevant. Evaluation of the patient's teaching must be seen in the context of the full cardiac rehabilitation service offered.

SUMMARY OF ESSENTIALS

Assessment of needs

In this chapter, the need for a proper assessment of the patient's and family's information needs before attempting to educate them about the recovery from a myocardial infarction has been stressed. In common with other areas of nursing care, the emphasis is on the needs of the individual. A prepared text for each patient who has had a heart attack will, however, appear impersonal and reduce the effectiveness of the teaching.

Communication

Patient education obviously relies on good communication between the patient, family and the health professional and some points are worth highlighting. Repetition of information at various stages is essential because of the patient and family's reduced ability to absorb information. Artinian (1989) describes how nurses may convey up to 65% of information in means other than verbal (e.g. by posture, gestures, facial expression and tone of voice) so the way in which something is said is as important as what is said. Explanations need to be as simple as possible in language that the patient and family can understand, avoiding the use of jargon. In some instances, the most effective interactions will be where the nurse speaks less than the patient.

Written information

The poor absorption of verbal information given to patients, especially during hospitalisation, has long been recognised (Conroy and Mulcahy, 1985). Therefore it is essential for the patient and his or her family to be supplied with written information. Patients may receive booklets from varying sources, from those produced by national organisations to those produced by staff within the hospital. Assessment of the usefulness of such literature often only goes as far as the content. The question of how readable and how understandable the information will be is often overlooked. This is of particular concern when considering the importance of patient leaflets in the total education of the patient and, from a financial point of view, the high level of resources spent on producing such literature. The importance of making written prose as readable as possible has been recognised for several years (Swanson, 1948). This recognition has led to the development of various readability formulae to assess the reading difficulty of written material Fry's readability graph (Fry, 1977) and the Gunning fog test cited by Albert and Chadwick (1992). Conroy and Mulcahy (1985) assessed written literature for cardiac patients using Fry's readability formula and found disturbingly that half the patients attending the hospital would only be able to read or understand 20% of the available literature. The essential point when preparing an information leaflet for patients it that must be assessed for content, readability, attractiveness and correct use of syntax (Albert and Chadwick, 1992). Dixon and Park (1990) correctly argue that, as the emphasis on patient education has increased, so have the expectations of the patient to understand information; written information must therefore meet this need.

REFERENCES

Albert, T., Chadwick, S. (1992). How readable are practice leaflets? *British Medical Journal*, **305**: 1266–1268.

Artinian, N. T. (1989). Family member perceptions of a cardiac surgery event. *Focus on Critical Care*, **16**(4): 301–308.

Chan, V. (1990). Content areas for cardiac teaching: patients' perceptions of the importance of teaching content after myocardial infarction. *Journal of Advanced Nursing*, **15**: 1139–1145.

Conroy, R. M., Mulchahy, R. (1985). Readability of literature written for cardiac patients. *Clinical Cardiology*, **8**: 104–106.

Daniels, L. (1989). Road to recovery. *Intensive Care Nursing*, **5**: 19–24.

Department of Health (1991). *The Patient's Charter. Raising the Standards*. HMSO, London.

Department of Health (1992). *Health of the Nation. Strategu for Health*. HMSO, London

Department of Health (1989). *A Strategy for Nursing. Report og the Steering Committee for the Department of Health Nursing Divide*. HMSO, London.

Dixon, E. and Park, R. (1990). Do patients understand written health information? *Nursing Outlook*, **38** (6): 278–281.

Fry, E. (1977). Fry's readability graph: clarification's, validity, and extension to level 17. *Journal of Reading*, **December**: 242–252.

Jacobsen, B. S. *et al.* (1992.) Why me? Causal thinking, affect, and expectations in myocardial infarction patients. *Journal of Cardiovascular Nursing*, 6(2): 57–65.

Johnson J. L., Morse J. M. (1990). Regaining control: the process of adjustment after myocardial infarction. *Heart and Lung*, **19**(2): 126–135.

Lowery B. J. (1991) Psychological stress, denial and myocardial infarction outcomes. *Image: Journal of Nursing Scholarship*, **23**(1): 51–55.

Lowery B. J. (1992) Attention versus avoidance: attributional search and denial after myocardial infarction. *Heart and Lung*, **21** (6): 523–528.

Lipetz, M. J. *et al.* (1990) What is wrong with patient education programmes? *Nursing Outlook*, **38** (4): 184–189.

Malan, S. S. (1992) Psychological adjustment following MI: current views and nursing implications. *Journal of Cardiovascular Nursing*, **6**(4): 57–70.

Marshall, J., Penchofer, S., Lleullyn, J. *et al.* (1986). Structured postoperative teaching and knowledge and compliance of patients who had coronary artery bypass surgery. *Heart and Lung*, **15**: 333–336.

Miller P., Wickoff, R., Garrett, M.J. *et al.* (1990) Regimen compliance two years after myocardial infarction. *Nursing research*, **39** (6): 333–336.

Moyniham, M (1984). Assessing the educational needs of post myocardial infarction patients. *Nursing Clinics of North America*, **19**(3): 441–447.

Nyamathi, A. M. (1990). Assessing the coping status of spouses of critically ill cardiac patients: a theoretically based approach. *Journal of Cardiovascular Nursing*, **5** (1): 1–12.

Penckofer S., Llewellyn J (1989) Adherence to risk factor instructions one year following coronary bypass surgery. *Journal of Cardiovascular Nursing*, **3** (3): 10–24.

Russell GC(1993) The role of denial in clinical practice. *Journal of Advanced Nursing*, **18**: 938–940.

Shearck K.A. (1992) Coping with acute myocardial infarction. *Heart and Lung* , **21**(4): 327–334.

Steele, J. M., Ruzicki, D. (1987). An evaluation of the effectiveness of cardiac teaching during hospitalisation. *Heart and Lung*, **16** (3): 306–311.

Swanson CE (1948) Readability and readership: a controlled experiment. *Journalism Quarterly*, **21**: 339–343.

Wallace, p., Joshi, M., C Wingett, C. *et al.* (1985) Nurses' perceptions of patients needs for information and their concerns in an English coronary care unit. *Intensive Care Nursing*, **1**: 84–91.

Wilson-Barnett J (1984) Alleviating stress for hospitalised patients. *International Review of Applied Psychology*, **33** (6), 493–503.

13.

PATIENT REHABILITATION

Interest in cardiac rehabilitation services has increased in recent years. This interest has grown from two sources: the patients and their families who seek information and guidance in their recovery from cardiac illness, and the care professionals who want to offer a complete service to patients to influence their long-term recovery.

This is reflected in the gradual increase in the availability of cardiac rehabilitation groups in the country. However, the situation is often dependent upon where the patient lives as to what service, if any, is offered. Horgan *et al.* (1992) in their report to the British Cardiac Society identified 92 centres supplying such a service. This accounted for less than 50% of Health Authorities in the country at that time. It is hoped that this situation will improve.

DEFINITION

The often quoted definition provided by the World Health Organisation cited by Deavin (1984) is succinct:

> 'The sum of activities required to ensure the best possible physical, mental and social conditions so that the patient may, by his [or her] own efforts, achieve and maintain their optimum state of health.'

The key phrases in this definition are 'sum of activities' and 'by his or her own efforts'. This acknowledges that cardiac rehabilitation is a multidisciplinary service to help patients regain control of their lives and take responsibility for their health. Cardiac rehabilitation will mean different things in different centres: from support groups in one area to long-term supervised exercise programmes in another. Cardiac rehabilitation programmes should not just be viewed as exercise groups for patients. While it is acknowledged that exercise is an essential and integral part of any rehabilitation programme, it is only a part of the total service. The patient who has regained a sufficient level of physical fitness but is scared to walk out of his or her front door can not be considered to be rehabilitated.

In the following pages, I relate my experience of working in a cardiac rehabilitation environment, focusing particularly on the nursing interventions used in this environment for a patient who has suffered MI. This approach is by no means the only one. Many people are working with varying resources throughout the country to help patients following MI or cardiac surgery. Cardiac rehabilitation may perhaps then be defined as any intervention that helps the patient and family return to some degree of normality.

THE PATIENT

Jack was a 66-year-old married man who had suffered an inferior MI while travelling to his place of work. This experience had radically changed his image of himself as a fit and active man. After the admission period of 8 days, during which Jack had experienced no complications, he was discharged home. Jack had left an impression on the ward as a sensible, cooperative, if slightly impatient, man. He had been a 'good patient', the type of patient who progresses steadily along what is considered the routine recovery of a person following a MI

I had first met Jack on the day after his admission in my capacity as the Cardiac Rehabilitation Nurse. I found him a pleasant man who was slightly wary of my intention in coming to speak to him. I explained to him that my role was to help him in his recovery from his heart attack by ensuring that he understood what had happened to his heart to help him recognise any modifiable cardiac risk factors in his lifestyle and advise on changes that may be necessary. Jack was not overweight, he denied smoking, kept himself fairly active and did not recognise any high levels of stress in his life. This made his heart attack seem very unfair to him. He told me that he had been married for 31 years, had a son who was married and lived in Newcastle. Jack had served for 20 years in the Royal Navy and since being discharged in 1975, he had had various jobs and was currently employed as a senior storeman in a large electrical manufacturing company. At the conclusion of our first meeting, I gave Jack an information leaflet about recovery from heart attacks for him to read at his leisure. I explained I would see him again 2 days later to discuss any concerns or questions he might have. He gave the impression that he thought I could spend my time more usefully seeing other patients.

I visited Jack again 2 days later, he had no questions to ask and said he had read the information leaflet, which he said he felt was self-explanatory. I mentioned the Outpatient Cardiac Rehabilitation Programme to him and suggested that this might be an option that he could consider to help him fully recover from his heart attack. His response was polite but he obviously did not consider such a service suitable for him. This was the last time I saw Jack as an inpatient. On my next visit to the ward I was told he had been discharged an hour earlier. I did not feel that I had been of any great help to Jack but at least he had my contact number if he wished to talk to me. I telephoned him 2 weeks after his discharge and he assured me he was recovering well. Jack was a reminder of the fact that effective nursing care is only possible through negotiation and agreement between the nurse and patient.

It was therefore with some surprise 4 months later that I received a telephone call from Jack asking to see me. We made an appointment for 3 days later and, in our long discussion, Jack described the difficulties he had experienced since leaving hospital. His confidence in his physical capabilities had diminished to a large degree, he appeared to feel very isolated, saying that nobody understood what it was like and he felt he was increasing his amount of cigarette smoking. This last statement was a surprise because he had previously not revealed that he had smoked at all. He explained this by saying he had only smoked five cigarettes a day and thought this of little consequence. He was now, he said, smoking between 15 and 20 per day. This was a different Jack from the one I had met in the ward, he had lost the self-confidence he had shown previously, his posture was slightly bowed, his voice softer and he looked older. I had said very little during the interview and he seemed to appreciate the chance to talk. He remembered my mention of the Cardiac Rehabilitation Programme and we mutually agreed to his attending the group to see if this would be of help to him.

NURSING ASSESSMENT

Jack's nursing care was assessed using Orem's *Self Care Model of Nursing*. Orem (1985) describes self care as 'the practice of activities that individuals initiate and perform on their own behalf to maintain life, health and well-being'. This definition has close similarities to the previously stated definition of cardiac rehabilitation. Both definitions focus on the patient's own efforts and are centred on the whole person. This common acceptance of the patient's responsibility in both Orem's model and the Cardiac Rehabilitation Programme was one of the factors that formed the basis of the rationale of the selection of Orem's model in Jack's care. Other factors would be:

- The environment of care. Jack would be attending the hospital two, sometimes three times a week, and the nursing strategy would be to identify actions that he could do for himself in his home environment to continue his recovery, for example, exercise.
- The priority of care differed to that which existed when Jack was admitted to hospital. Then survival was the priority goal but this had now changed and Orem's emphasis on the well-being of the patient was highly relevant.
- Orem places high priority on the assessment of the patient being an on-going process and the need to work with the patient and his or her family. The nurse's role was to act as an educator, advisor and supporter. Jack had survived his heart attack and the nursing need now was to examine and alter how he survived.

Assessing Jack's need for care involved applying the information he offered to the identified universal self care needs. Jack had returned to me displaying a high level of anxiety about his health and ability to live life in the manner he wished. This was Jack's individual definition of normal life and needs some further description here.

Jack's years in the armed services had left him with a disciplined attitude to life, he remained physically active, his main interests being walking and to running a local 11-year-olds' football team. He was 1 year past retirement age but had been allowed to continue his employment, which he greatly enjoyed and valued. He had a mistrust of illness and saw his lifestyle as his right, owing to his taking care of himself throughout his life. The fact that he was smoking did not enter into this equation. It was obvious that Jack felt very isolated. In his social circle he was now not seen as the active healthy person he had always portrayed himself. He said he could not (maybe would not) seek support from his friends as they would not understand. He said it was as though he was the only person in the world to have had a heart attack.

Jack was willing to accept my assertion that he must look at methods to stop smoking. Coming from a generation where smoking was actively encouraged, he found this difficult and admitted openly that he enjoyed a cigarette. Jack's need for care was based on the fact that his heart attack had rocked the very foundations of his life. The first four of Orem's universal self care needs were not a problem in Jack's case. He had sufficient intake of air, water and food and had no problems with elimination. The deviation existed in his ability to maintain a balance between rest and activity owing to his lack of confidence in his physical abilities.

Jack had a high element of physical demand in his social and work life but had difficulty in coping with those demands. No physical infirmity was present to influence this. Jack's isolation and the lack of knowledge about his heart attack and recovery had resulted in a deviation in his ability to maintain a balance between solitude and social interaction. This had placed a further burden of anxiety on Jack. His ability to cope with this demand and achieve self care would depend on him taking a more realistic view of himself and how he portrayed himself in the future. Jack's smoking habit could be seen as an imbalance in the prevention of hazards to himself. Although he expressed agreement to this, his determination was not very convincing. To achieve self care in this respect (i.e. to give up smoking) he would need extended support beyond that would be offered through the Cardiac Rehabilitation Programme.

His final deviation from self-care was in the last category – to be normal. His reaction to his heart attack had prevented him from achieving this state. Jack could define 'normal' as being able to live his life in the active manner he had done so before his heart problem. This was generally a realistic objective, these activities were within his capabilities and, given his motivated attitude apparent by his action in seeking help, he had great potential to achieve this.

PLANNING THE NURSING CARE

Jack had agreed to attend the Outpatient cardiac rehabilitation programme which was held in his local hospital. The aim of the programme was to address physical, psychological and lifestyle problems of the patient following MI or heart surgery. As already stated, Jack had little confidence in his ability to exercise. He was concerned that exercise would provoke the onset of another heart attack – 'a time bomb in my chest' he remarked. The nurse's role in his care was to provide supportive education. In the environment and situation in which care was delivered, there were no instances where the nurse could act as a wholly or compensatory agent for Jack. Actions were based on Orem's model to instil confidence in Jack to allow him to achieve his objectives.

The exercise component of his care offered a graduated exercise programme in a supervised environment with the attendance of nurses and physiotherapists. The exercises were of an aerobic nature and would be increased gradually over the 6 weeks that Jack would be attending the course.

Exercise in cardiac patients has been shown to be beneficial in several ways. Ewart et al. (1983) showed an increase in the patient's perception of their physical capacity following exercise. Kannel et al. (1985) showed a beneficial effect of moderate exercise in lowering atherosclerotic risk factors. Wenger and Alpert (1989) show lessened levels of depression, resumption of sexual activity and an earlier return to pre-illness social roles.

While being in a group situation with other patients who have been through a similar experience to himself, Jack would be able to gain peer support and reduce his feelings of isolation. Further interventions were planned to reduce Jack's feelings of anxiety.

The psychological effect on the recovery of a person following a MI is well recognized. Thompson *et al.* (1990) showed an increased satisfaction in the life and health of patients who had received counselling beginning during the admission phase. Jack would receive one-to-one counselling support, instruction in relaxation therapy, which has been shown to enhance the long-term outcome following MI in conjunction with exercise training (Dixhoorn, 1987).

Lastly, involvement in a group education programme was aimed at adjusting his life following MI and reducing any risk factors in his lifestyle. Jack's smoking was a relevant issue in this area. Reduction in his anxiety level was seen as a factor helping him to stop smoking but the need was also to look at the reasons why he smoked and to advise him on methods to control the cause rather than just tell him to stop.

Jack would attend the Cardiac Rehabilitation Programme twice weekly for a fixed period of 6 weeks. His condition and progress would be evaluated following each session by the multidisciplinary team working on the programme. It was envisaged that, as he progressed in the programme, work skills supervised by the occupational therapist would be introduced. This would allow him to simulate some of the physical elements of his job to prepare him to return to his employment.

The plan of care was agreed by Jack, and myself, and he attended the programme for the first time 1 week after seeing me.

NURSING INTERVENTION

Exercise

The nurse's role in supervising Jack during the exercise was to liaise closely with the physiotherapists who were responsible for prescribing the exercise programme. Monitoring Jack's condition was a nursing responsibility. This was achieved in several ways: on his arrival to each session, Jack and the Cardiac Rehabilitation Nurse would discuss his progress and general health and identify any problems that had occurred since he had previously attended the group. Baseline heart rate recording was taken, and further readings were taken during and after the exercise sessions for comparison. Jack's pulse was monitored during the exercise to ensure it kept within a range of 75% of an agreed maximum. This figure was the maximum heart rate achieved during Jack's exercise ECG test. Jack was instructed on how to take his own pulse to allow him to take some responsibility in this measurement. Blood-pressure recordings were taken before and after exercise. Any element of competition was discouraged strongly and Jack was instructed to sit out of the session if he felt any particular activity was beyond him. The importance of reporting any symptoms he may have suffered was also stressed. Here again he was taking a measure of responsibility.

At first, Jack was reticent about taking exercise. In the early sessions he was worried about getting out of breath and perspiring. He equated this with his experience during his heart attack. He would only feel safe if he had another member of staff working with him. After the first 2 weeks this began to change. He settled into the group and began to make acquaintances and required less overt supervision.

Psychological support

Jack initially had great difficulty with the group relaxation sessions, he found the whole experience very alien but agreed to persevere with the therapy. We had agreed to meet weekly to discuss his reaction to, and recovery from, his heart attack as a way of helping him to identify problems and learn coping strategies.

It was after three of these one-to-one sessions that Jack began to take an interest in and gain some benefit from the relaxation session. The sessions allowed Jack to talk about his heart attack. He discussed in full what had happened on the day, describing the pain, prospect of sudden death and the panic that ensued. On other occasions, he talked of his time following discharge up to the time when he made contact with me again. He tried to return to his former life and was shocked to discover the reduction in his stamina. He had become withdrawn, irritable and found sleeping difficult. My role was to listen, reflect, challenge and support him generally. I took great care to avoid telling him what he ought to do. Any change in his life had to be decided by him and thus owned by him to be effective.

Education

Jack involved himself enthusiastically in the educational and discussional sessions in the programme. As the weeks progressed he became increasingly active and was asking varied questions. The sessions were balanced to look equally at the issues of recovering from MI, and returning to normal life, and risk-factor modification. Jack was also referred to a counsellor who specialised in helping people to stop smoking.

EVALUATION OF NURSING CARE

Orem's model of nursing care stresses the need for the assessment process to be an ongoing one. It was by following this process that Jack's care was evaluated. The evaluation involved looking for evidence in Jack's behaviour that indicated that he was gradually achieving self-care in the areas that he had identified as being deficient because of the effect of his illness. Since Jack had set his own objectives when joining the rehabilitation programme, he was encouraged to continue his exercise and to attempt to stop smoking away from us in his home environment. His opinion of his progress had also to be considered. This added a subjective element to the evaluation that was highly relevant as one of his objectives was to be 'normal'.

Physically Jack progressed well through the programme. By the fifth week he displayed confidence in exercising with minimal supervision. He enjoyed the sessions and expressed verbally his satisfaction in his perceived improvement. He had started swimming and was enjoying taking regular walks. Occasionally his competitive nature would show and he needed reminding of his initial objectives. By the end of the 6-week programme he was exercising freely without symptoms and could be considered as having achieved self-care in this respect.

This degree of self-care was reflected in his mental attitude. He became more outgoing, his statements about life and himself were increasingly positive. He had also returned to many of his old social contacts and had made new ones during his time on the programme. He took an interest in the relaxation techniques and was given a tape to use at home.

In a more objective area of evaluation Jack had not, at the time of his completing the programme, stopped smoking. He had reduced his intake from 30 to 10 cigarettes/day. It is possible that his feeling of well-being made the warnings about the dangers of smoking less real to him. He had always said he had enjoyed a cigarette so his determination to stop was questionable. The difference now was that he had continued to smoke despite having been informed of, and experienced the dangers of, continuing to do so. It may be possible to argue perhaps that, in this context, although the nursing objectives had not been achieved, he had in fact achieved a form of self-care. This is a salutary reminder that when promoting self-care and the patient's responsibility for his or her health, we cannot always expect the outcome to meet our own preferred objectives.

SUMMARY OF ESSENTIALS

Criteria for attending a rehabilitation group

In the previous section, the essential role of planning and of setting objectives for a patient attending a cardiac rehabilitation course has been discussed. By using this approach, the programme can be adapted to meet the individual patient's needs. This has the benefit of making the programme available to a wider number of patients. For example, patients who, for whatever reason, are unable to take part in the exercise component of the programme, should not be excluded because they may gain benefit from the educational component of the programme. The beneficial effects of peer support obtained from the group environment should not be underestimated.

Age is sometimes used as a factor for excluding patients from rehabilitation programmes. The author would argue strongly against this and advocates that each patient should be assessed on his individual merits. The medical criteria for patients' inclusion in programmes will differ according to the local policies. The policy used in the author's unit will therefore be discussed.

Patients who have suffered a MI may attend 2 weeks after their MI provided that they have achieved a negative exercise ECG on a modified Bruce Protocol. Patients whose exercise ECG is positive and are to be treated medically may attend on the doctor's recommendation. Patients who have undergone cardiac surgery may attend after 4 weeks. This allows a period of convalescence and promotes healing of the sternum. Patients with other cardiac conditions such as arrhythmias, left ventricular failure or chronic angina may attend following referral from, and discussion with, medical staff.

Patient safety

Obviously the safety of a patient is of paramount importance. The beneficial effects of exercise in cardiac patients is generally recognised (Fletcher, 1984; Diethrich, 1987; Bethell, 1990). However, it is essential that any exercise programme is prescribed by adequately trained personnel, i.e. physiotherapists or exercise physiologists. Examples of exercise circuits abound (Turner, 1986).

The nurse has a major role in the multidisciplinary team in ensuring the safety of the patient during exercise, firstly in the selection of patients. In addition to adhering to the agreed protocol, the nurse has the advantage of having followed the patient through the acute stage of the illness. The nurse will therefore have a knowledge of the events during the patient's hospital stay and will have developed an initial rapport with the patient. This, along with the initial assessment processes, can identify any early problems that may occur during exercise, e.g. very competitive patients who need to be discouraged and guided, or patients who have other health problems such as musculoskeletal problems where high-impact exercises should be avoided. The graduated nature of the exercises should also be stressed to allow the patient to ease themselves into the programme gradually. Facilities for cardiac monitoring may be available in some units, although this will depend on resources available. Cardiopulmonary resuscitation equipment should be available within the unit, and staff trained in basic and advanced life-support techniques.

Duration of course

The duration of cardiac rehabilitation courses will vary according to the individual centre's policy and will depend on the stated objectives of that programme. However, there is an argument for offering courses of a set duration. If the stated aim is to help the patient make the transition from the cardiac patient back to the normal person again, one must be careful not to supplant one form of dependency upon hospital staff for dependency on the rehabilitation staff. By offering a course of 6 weeks, a stepping stone is provided for the patient to return to normal.

Consideration of individual cases is essential in this and obviously there will be some patients who will benefit from a longer period on a rehabilitation programme; however, one must retain sight of the need to match actions and objectives. This approach, however, may not be appropriate for other centres whose objectives differ e.g. centres who offer long-term exercise programmes for an expected physical benefit.

Psychological care

Psychological care of the patient following a MI is a common theme that runs through all activities in the cardiac rehabilitation process. In outpatient cardiac rehabilitation groups, exercise instruction and education have a great role in providing this support. However, two other factors may also be considered: the instruction of patients in methods of relaxation, and meeting a group of people who know exactly what they have experienced.

The instruction of patients in methods of relaxation with the aim of giving the patient guidance on dealing with life stresses is another intervention to try to help the patient to regain control. Several studies have suggested the benefit of relaxation training following a cardiac event (Johnston and Lo, 1983; Dixhoorn et al. 1987).

The peer support that can be gained from attending a regular rehabilitation class can be one of the great benefits for patients. The isolation felt by many cardiac patients following discharge can be particularly acute. They have moved fairly rapidly from a sudden situation where death has been a possibility to a return to their home environment, distancing themselves from the hospital and carers in which they had placed so much trust. To quote Davidson (1989):

'Both patient and family may leave the hospital with an inappropriate appraisal of causes of the event and with pessimistic assessments of prognosis, often leading to unwarranted fears and limitations of activities'.

Situations like this may deny the patient the opportunity to discuss his or her feelings about his or her cardiac illness and his recovery. Friends may ask the question 'How are you?' but may have problems in dealing with the patient who replies and reveals his or her true feelings and fears about recovery. The patient is generally required to respond 'I'm fine'. Therefore meeting people who know exactly what it is like, who have experienced similar fears, is of tremendous value to both the patient and his family.

EDUCATION

This has been discussed in the previous chapter; however, regarding the educational content, there should be an equal balance between risk-factor modification and advice on returning to normal following or living with heart disease.

The patient's family

The involvement of a patient's family in all aspects of the cardiac rehabilitation process is essential. Nyamathi (1990) and Gillis et al. (1990) among others have recognised the crucial role played by family in the patient's long-term recovery. Thompson et al. (1990) shows increased satisfaction with life in the 6 months following a MI when education and psychological support were offered to both the patient and their spouse. In the outpatient cardiac rehabilitation setting, difficulties may arise since it is often difficult for partners to attend because of other commitments, the ongoing perception of it just being an exercise group may also make the partner feel that it is not appropriate for them to attend. This is an intervention that must be offered jointly to both the patient and family. The emerging role of cardiac support groups in offering a supportive social environment to cardiac patients and their families may also be of benefit.

Evaluation

Evaluation of a cardiac rehabilitation programme is a controversial issue. Expected benefit in reduction of mortality of patients following a MI has not been shown. Despite meta-analysis by Oldridge *et al.* (1988) suggesting a 20% reduction in mortality and O'Connor *et al.* (1989), the position remains inconclusive. Therefore cardiac rehabilitation, in common with many other nursing interventions, must rely on the subjectiveness of its nature, allowing the patient to work towards what he or she defines as being normal life. This means that each patient will have a different end-point. This situation makes objective measurement of cardiac rehabilitation extremely difficult. Therefore it is in the areas of quality of life and patient well-being that cardiac rehabilitation is expected to have a beneficial effect. This is now generally accepted and well supported by numerous studies (Conn *et al.*, 1992; Campbell, 1993; Wenger and Alpert, 1989).

Since current Government emphasis is on improving quality of services for patients, cardiac rehabilitation is in a prime position to assert itself as a necessary and effective intervention in the total recovery of the cardiac patient, provided that it maintains a clear idea of what it is hoping to achieve for each patient.

CARDIAC REHABILITATION EXERCISE CIRCUIT

The exercise session lasts approximately 1 hour and contains three main components:warm up (including stretches),. circuit exercises (aerobic), and cool down, including stretches.

Warm up

This lasts approximately 10–15 minutes and is a group session with a similar routine every session so that the patients may use this at home. The stretches are upper and lower limb and each stretch should have a 10–15 second hold.

Circuit

A maximum of 12 patients per circuit should be allowed. The following exercises are used:

- Step-ups.
- Trampette.
- Stepper.
- Exercise bike.
- Sit-to-stand-ups.
- Treadmill.
- Skipping.
- Marching.
- Bouncing ball around obstacles.

The circuit exercises start at 30–45 second duration and progress to 75 seconds. The rest in between exercises is timed and is approximately 30–60 seconds, according to the group's abilities. The circuit should contain aerobic exercises and last for a minimum of 20 minutes to maintain the patient's pulse within their training range. If appropriate, strengthening exercises can be used at the end of the circuit before the cool-down period. To allow healing of the sternum, weight-bearing arm exercises should not be started until 6 weeks after the operation.

Cool down

This time can be used for coordination exercises. It should last 10 minutes and includes stretches similar to the warm up.

REFERENCES

Bethell, H. (1991). Does exercise prolong life after a coronary? *Cardiology in Practice*, **8** (6): 9–11.

Campbell, J. (1993). How necessary is cardiac rehabilitation. *Professional Nurse*, **8** (5): 279–283.

Conn, V.S. Taylor, S.G., Casey, B. *et al.* (1992). Cardiac rehabilitation program participation and outcomes after myocardial infarction. *Rehabilitation Nursing*, **17:** 58–62.

Davidson, D.M. (1989). Family and sexual adjustments after cardiac events. *Quality of Life and Cardiovascular Care*, **Summer:** 66–79.

Diethrich, E.B. (1987). Condemned: is there an alternative for the patient with severe coronary artery disease? *Critical Care Nursing*, **9** (4), 8–13.

Deavin, J. (1984). Rehabilitation following myocardial infarction. *Nursing*, **25:** 740–742.

Dixhoorn, J. (1987). Cardiac events after myocardial infarction: possible effect of relaxation therapy. *European Heart Journal*, **8:** 1210–1214.

Ewart, C. K., Barr-Taylor, C., Rees, L.B. *et al.* (1983). Effects of early post-myocardial infarction exercise testing on self perception and subsequent physical activity. *American Journal of Cardiology*, **51:** 1076–1080.

Fletcher, G.F. (1984) Long-term exercise in coronary artery disease and other chronic disease states. *Heart and Lung*, **13** (1): 28-44.

Gillis C. L., Neihaus, J., Hauck, W. *et al.* (1990) Improving family functioning after cardiac surgery: a randomised trial. *Heart and Lung*, **19** (6): 648–659.

Horgan, P., Bethell, H., Carson, P., *et al.* (1992).Working pay report on cardiac rehabilitation. *British Heart Journal*, **67**: 412–418.

Johnston, D.W., Lo, C.R. (1983). The effects of cardiovascular feedback and relaxation on angina pectoris. *Behavioural Psychotherapy*, **11**: 257–264.

Kannel ,W.B., Wilson, P., Blair, F.N. *et al.* (1985). Epidemiological assessment of the role of physical activity and fitness in the development of cardiovascular disease. *American Heart Journal*, **109** (4): 876–885.

Nyamathi, A.M. (1990). Assessing the coping status of spouses of critically ill cardiac patients: a theoretically based approach. *Journal of Cardiovascular Nursing*, **5** (1): 1–12.

O'Connor, G. T. *et al.* (1989). An overview of randomized trials of rehabilitation with exercise after myocardial infarction. *Circulation*, **80** (2): 234–244.

Oldridge, N. B. *et al.* (1988). Cardiac rehabilitation after myocardial infarction. Combined experience of randomized clinical trials. *Journal of the American Medical Association*, **260** (7): 945–950.

Orem, D. (1985). *Nursing: Concepts of Practice*, 3rd edn. McGraw-Hill, Maidenhead.

Thompson, D. R. *et al.* (1990). In-hospital counselling for firs-time myocardial infarction patient and spouses: effects on satisfaction. *Journal of Advanced Nursing*, **15**: 1064–1069.

Turner, S.C. (1986). Exercise training in a community sports centre. *Physiotherapy* **72** (5): 229–233.

Wenger, N. K., Alpert, J. S. (1989). Rehabilitation of the coronary patient in 1989. *Archive of International Medicine*, **149**: 1504–1506.

INDEX